Evidence-Based Practices for Eating Disorder Treatment

Jennifer Schulz
Ashland University, USA

IGI Global
Scientific Publishing
Publishing Tomorrow's Research Today

Vice President of Editorial	Melissa Wagner
Director of Acquisitions	Mikaela Felty
Director of Book Development	Jocelynn Hessler
Production Manager	Mike Brehm
Cover Design	Jose Rosado

Published in the United States of America by
IGI Global Scientific Publishing
701 East Chocolate Avenue
Hershey, PA, 17033, USA
Tel: 717-533-8845 | Fax: 717-533-7115
Website: https://www.igi-global.com E-mail: cust@igi-global.com

Library of Congress Cataloging-in-Publication Data

Names: Schulz, Jennifer, 1990- editor
Title: Evidence-based practices for eating disorder treatment / edited by Jennifer Schulz.
Description: Hershey, PA : IGI Global Scientific Publishing, [2026] | Includes bibliographical references and index. | Summary: "This book aims to provide a summary of eating disorder interventions, and their effects in various populations. Research related to eating disorder treatment modalities is limited"-- Provided by publisher.
Identifiers: LCCN 2025020196 (print) | LCCN 2025020197 (ebook) | ISBN 9798337306643 h/c | ISBN 9798337306650 s/c | ISBN 9798337306667 ebook
Subjects: LCSH: Eating disorders--Treatment--Research | Evidence-based medicine
Classification: LCC RC552.E18 E947 2026 (print) | LCC RC552.E18 (ebook)
LC record available at https://lccn.loc.gov/2025020196
LC ebook record available at https://lccn.loc.gov/2025020197

British Cataloguing in Publication Data
A Cataloguing in Publication record for this book is available from the British Library.

Table of Contents

Preface

As both a licensed social worker who stays active in clinical practice, and a university professor preparing the next generation of mental health professionals for clinical practice, I have a vested interest in eating disorder treatment. After all, eating disorders are diagnosable mental health disorders. Despite this fact, I have been surprised to find that there is a lack of comprehensive textbooks related to eating disorder treatment. A quick Internet search does reveal some textbooks on this topic, but there are limitations. For instance, many books are outdated, published longer than 10 years ago. In addition, these texts are not entirely comprehensive. For instance, they may only cover psychotherapy methods used in eating disorder treatment, while ignoring complementary treatments, such as nutrition counseling. Or, they may provide information on treatment, without introducing readers to background information about eating disorder diagnostic criteria and risk factors, which I would argue is germane to a textbook on evidence-based eating disorder treatment.

With the above in mind, I was driven to prepare a textbook on evidence-based eating disorder treatments, appropriate for a wide range of audiences. Given the paucity of texts on this topic, it's essential that such a book be appropriate for a wide range of professionals who may become involved in eating disorder treatment. As such, this text is appropriate not only for mental health clinicians, including counselors, social workers, psychologists, and marriage and family therapists; it's also suitable for medical staff, including psychiatrists and nurses working in psychiatric care.

Textbooks on eating disorder treatment are an essential component of the curriculum for university-level training programs for all of the previously mentioned professions. For example, experts have recommended that psychotherapists should be required to obtain a minimum level of competence in eating disorder treatment, to include assessment and diagnosis, intervention strategies, nutritional and medical factors, interdisciplinary collaboration, and levels of care (Spotts-De Lazzer & Muhlheim, 2016). While research on competency levels in professionals is limited, what little research is available demonstrates that clinicians are not entirely competent, especially when it comes to eating disorder assessment. For example, in a study of clinical social workers, MacCaughelty (2023) found that 42.4% of social workers did not assess for eating disorders during the intake process. Given the importance of eating disorder assessment and intervention, the lack of available print resources on this topic, and the high proportion of clinicians not assessing for eating disorder symptoms, the current textbook fills a critical gap. Below, I will describe the overall layout and content of the textbook, to provide instructors and readers with a comprehensive overview of what to expect from this text.

CONTENT AND LAYOUT

This textbook is intended to be comprehensive, covering a wide range of topics related to eating disorder assessment and treatment. It is divided into three overarching sections to partition the content. The first section includes three chapters that form the foundation of understanding concepts related to eating disorder assessment and treatment. The text begins with a chapter that describes eating disorder diagnoses as they appear in the 5th edition, text revised version of the *Diagnostic and Statistical Manual of Mental Disorders*. Understanding diagnostic criteria for eating disorders is an essential component of eating disorder assessment, and as such is a central feature of this book. The first chapter also discusses evidence-based assessment tools that can be utilized to screen for eating disorders and assist with making diagnoses based on DSM-5-TR criteria. The next chapter discusses eating disorder risk factors and epidemiology, which serves two purposes. First, it's essential to understand the root causes of eating disorders, as these causes may inform interventions. Second, understanding prevalence rates of eating disorders can be helpful for the differential diagnosis process, as a clinician must consider base rates of a disorder when making a diagnosis (Finn, 2009). The first section finishes with the third chapter, which addresses the history of eating disorder treatment, to create a context for the rest of the text.

The next section of the textbook covers eating disorder treatment modalities and includes chapters 4-10, making it the most substantial section of the text. This section begins with a systematic review of eating disorder treatment modalities. This systematic review was conducted specifically for inclusion in this text, to ensure that readers have a comprehensive understanding of the existing literature on eating disorder treatment. It is intended to provide an all-encompassing, non-biased overview of eating disorder interventions. After this initial chapter, various specific therapeutic modalities that may be used in eating disorder treatment are discussed in detail. Some chapters describe specific approaches, such as psychodynamic therapy, whereas others are broader, covering family-based or group-based interventions.

Finally, section three of the text covers additional considerations in eating disorder treatment. Level of care, which is an essential component of treatment planning, has its own chapter. This section also addresses other topics relevant to treatment planning, including who is on the eating disorder treatment team, as well as gaps in knowledge and cultural considerations in eating disorder treatment. The text concludes with a quick reference section, where readers can locate pertinent information related to key concepts in eating disorder treatment.

INTENDED AUDIENCE

This text is written with several audiences in mind. First, it is appropriate for a variety of mental health professionals, including social workers, psychologists, marriage and family therapists, and counselors. It is also appropriate for medical providers, including psychiatrists and psychiatric nurses. The latter could include both registered nurses and nurse practitioners working in psychiatric settings. All of these professionals play a central role in eating disorder assessment and intervention, and as such, they can also benefit from this text.

With that in mind, professionals already working in the field might use this text as a reference. For instance, they may refer to it when completing an assessment, or they might visit a specific chapter to refresh their knowledge of a particular therapeutic modality. Beyond use in professional settings, this text is also appropriate for use in graduate school programs in social work, psychology, nursing, and marriage and family therapy. Medical schools might also include this text in their curriculum to prepare students for specialization in psychiatry.

While this text is intended for graduate students and professional audiences, it may also be suitable for upper-division undergraduate courses. For instance, psychology or social work students may take a class on eating disorder treatment as part of a specialization, or perhaps as a senior year elective. With mastery of earlier coursework, particularly related to abnormal psychology and counseling skills, students can successfully engage with the material in this text.

AUTHOR'S QUALIFICATIONS

As the author of this text, I am passionate about eating disorder prevention, treatment, and intervention. I am a licensed social worker with a master's degree in social work, with a clinical focus, and a doctoral degree in psychology. I am both a practicing clinician, with years of experience as a crisis therapist, and a university faculty member. I have taught courses on human behavior and abnormal psychology, and I have written curriculum related to eating disorder assessment and treatment. I bring a unique perspective to a text of this topic, as both a practicing clinician and a faculty member committed to delivering high-quality curriculum to the next generation of clinicians.

In addition to my clinical and teaching experience, I am an avid researcher. I have recently written a textbook on research methods for the social sciences. I have also taught courses on research methods, and I am passionate about the importance of evidence-based practices. My research interests focus on eating disorder treatment and prevention. The current text combines my passion for eating disorder awareness with my skills as a researcher, and I hope it will help readers to develop a mastery of evidence-based practices for people living with eating disorders.

ACKNOWLEDGMENTS

Thank you to my colleagues at Ashland University, and specifically in the Department of Psychology, Social Work, and Criminal Justice, for supporting me in taking on this project. Thank you also to my early career mentors at Mount Vernon Nazarene University, including Dr. Jean Ollis. A huge thanks also goes out to my students at both Ashland University and Mount Vernon Nazarene University for motivating me to be the best educator I can; to my son Johnathan, for reminding me that little eyes are always watching; and to my husband, Troy, for supporting all of my dreams.

REFERENCES

Finn, S. E. (2009). Incorporating base rate information in daily clinical decision making. In Butcher, J. N. (Ed.), *Oxford handbook of personality assessment* (pp. 140–149). Oxford University Press., DOI: 10.1093/oxfordhb/9780195366877.013.0008

MacCaughelty, C. R. (2023). Eating disorder mental health literacy: A national survey of clinical social workers in the United States. *Journal of Social Work : JSW*, *23*(2), 300–316. DOI: 10.1177/14680173221144217

Spotts-De Lazzer, A., & Muhlheim, L. (2016). Eating disorders and scope of competence for outpatient psychotherapists. *Practice Innovations (Washington, D.C.)*, *1*(2), 89–104. DOI: 10.1037/pri0000021

Introduction

Eating disorders represent some of the most complex and challenging conditions in the field of mental health. Characterized by persistent disturbances in eating behavior and body image, these disorders—such as anorexia nervosa, bulimia nervosa, and binge-eating disorder—often involve significant physical, emotional, and social consequences. While once considered rare, eating disorders are now recognized as prevalent across diverse populations and developmental stages, with growing awareness of their presence in individuals of all genders, races, ages, and socioeconomic backgrounds.

In the chapters that follow, this textbook aims to offer a comprehensive exploration of evidence-based treatments for eating disorders, integrating psychotherapeutic, behavioral, relational, and systemic approaches. Chapters include critical discussions of psychodynamic therapy, interpersonal psychotherapy, dialectical behavior therapy, cognitive-behavioral therapy, family-based interventions, and emerging modalities such as neuromodulation and emotion-focused approaches. Each treatment model is examined through its theoretical foundation, empirical support, clinical applications, and limitations, offering students and mental health professionals a nuanced understanding of the multidimensional nature of eating disorder treatment.

Through clinical case studies, research reviews, and practical considerations for implementation, this volume aims to bridge the gap between research and practice, which has been identified as critical for improving services provided to patients with eating disorder diagnoses. Readers will be equipped not only to recognize the symptoms and systemic impacts of eating disorders but also to critically evaluate and apply treatment models in ethically informed and culturally responsive ways. Ultimately, this book is designed to support the development of competent, compassionate clinicians who are prepared to navigate the evolving landscape of eating disorder treatment. Given the consequences of these disorders, as well as the lack of trained professionals, it is essential for those entering the behavioral health field to develop competence in this area.

Section 1

Foundations of Eating Disorder Assessment and Treatment

Chapter 1
Eating Disorder Assessment Utilizing the DSM-5-TR

ABSTRACT

This chapter introduces readers to the eating disorder diagnoses in the Feeding and Eating Disorders chapter of the DSM-5-TR. Each eating disorder diagnosis in this chapter is described in detail, giving readers a thorough understanding of the eating disorders that may be diagnosed in clinical practice. Readers will be exposed to the diagnostic criteria for the various eating disorders, preparing them to make a diagnosis in clinical practice. The chapter also covers valid, reliable diagnostic tools that can be used to assist with making an eating disorder diagnosis.

INTRODUCTION

In clinical settings in the United States, *The Diagnostic and Statistical Manual of Mental Disorders*, 5th edition, text revision (DSM-5-TR), is used to diagnose eating disorders. The DSM-5-TR describes multiple distinct disorders, in a chapter titled "Feeding and Eating Disorders." What these disorders have in common is a disturbance in eating behaviors, which leads to distress and dysfunction (American Psychiatric Association, 2022). Understanding DSM-5-TR disorders and their respective diagnostic criteria is essential for professionals engaged in eating disorder assessment

DOI: 10.4018/979-8-3373-0664-3.ch001

and intervention. It's critical for professionals to recognize that there is not one universal presentation associated with an eating disorder. Instead, there are various distinct disorders, each with its own symptoms and corresponding treatment needs. In this chapter, the various eating disorders in the DSM-5-TR are described in detail; readers will also be introduced to psychometrically sound assessment tools that can be used in clinical practice.

TYPES OF EATING DISORDERS IN THE DSM-5-TR

The term "eating disorder" probably evokes a certain image in the mind. Perhaps, for example, you think of someone who severely restricts calories because of an intense fear of gaining weight. While this certainly aligns with anorexia nervosa, the reality is that this is not the only presentation of an eating disorder. There are several eating disorders defined in the DSM-5-TR, and they vary significantly in their presentation. For instance, some eating disorders involve a disturbance in body image, whereas others do not (American Psychiatric Association, 2022). The specific eating disorders and their distinct diagnostic features are described below in more detail.

Anorexia Nervosa

Anorexia nervosa is often regarded as the most serious of the eating disorders, based on its mortality rate, which is higher than for all other psychiatric disorders aside from opioid use disorder. Individuals with anorexia nervosa have an intense fear of gaining weight and engage in self-starvation, leading to severe weight loss and a significantly low body weight (Guarda, 2023). To be diagnosed with anorexia nervosa, a person must reduce their calorie intake below what is required, to the point that their body weight is less that what is minimally normal. They must also have an extreme fear of weight gain or ongoing behavior that prevents weight gain, even when their weight remains low. Finally, a person must experience a disturbance in their perception of body weight and shape, preoccupation with body weight and shape when evaluating the self, or failure to recognize the severity of their low body weight (American Psychiatric Association, 2022).

There are two primary types of anorexia nervosa: the restricting type and the binge-eating/purging type. As these names suggest, the restricting type involves achieving a low body weight by dieting, fasting, or excessive exercise, without any recurrent episodes of binge-eating or purging over the previous three months. On the other hand, the binge-eating/purging subtype involves presentations in which a person has engaged in recurrent episodes of binge-eating or purging over the previous three months. Anorexia can further be specified as mild, moderate, severe, or extreme, based on one's body mass index. For instance, an individual with a BMI equal to or above 17 is classified as having mild anorexia nervosa, whereas someone with a BMI below 15 is classified as having extreme anorexia nervosa (American Psychiatric Association, 2022). See Table 1 below for an overview of anorexia nervosa diagnostic criteria.

Table 1. Anorexia nervosa diagnostic criteria

General Diagnostic Criteria
• Restricting calorie intake in such a manner that body weight falls below what is minimally normal • Extreme fear of weight gain or behavior that prevents weight gain, despite being at significantly low body weight • Distorted perception of one's weight or shape, excessive influence placed one one's body weight or shape when evaluating the self, or failure to recognize the severity of low body weight
Severity Specifiers
• Mild: BMI greater than or equal to 17 • Moderate: BMI of 16-16.99 • Severe: BMI of 15-15.99 • Extreme: BMI under 15

continued on following page

Table 1. Continued

Other Specifiers
• Restricting type: A person has not engaging in repeated episodes of being-eating or purging within last 3 months and has achieved weight loss primarily by dieting, fasting, or using excessive exercise. • Binge-eating/purging type: A person has engaged in repeated episode of binge-eating or purging during the previous three months. • In partial remission: After previously meeting all three of the general diagnostic criteria noted above, a person has no longer met the first criterion noted above, but has met one of the other two. • In full remission: A person previously met full criteria for anorexia nervosa but has not met any of the general diagnostic criteria above for a sustained period.

Bulimia Nervosa

As can be the case with anorexia nervosa, bulimia nervosa involves a fixation on body weight and shape when evaluating oneself; however, bulimia is distinct from anorexia in several ways. First, individuals with bulimia nervosa experience recurrent episodes of binge eating, during which time they consume much larger amounts of food than most people would consume over a particular period of time, such as a two-hour window. During binge episodes, individuals living with bulimia nervosa lose control over the amount of food that is consumed, to the point that they are unable to stop eating. Alongside binges, individuals with bulimia nervosa engage in inappropriate compensatory behaviors to rid the body of excess calories and prevent weight gain. Such behaviors include forced vomiting, misusing laxatives or diuretics, fasting, or engaging in excessive exercise. A person must engage in this pattern of binging and purging at least weekly for three months to be diagnosed, and their self-evaluation must be overly influenced by body weight and shape (American Psychiatric Association, 2022).

As is the case with anorexia nervosa, there are severity specifiers of mild, moderate, severe, and extreme for bulimia nervosa. The disorder is labeled as mild when inappropriate compensatory behaviors occur on average of one to three times per week and moderate when such episodes occur an average of four to seven times per week. Severe presentations of bulimia nervosa involve an average of eight to 13 weekly episodes of inappropriate compensatory behaviors, and extreme presentations involve an average of 14 or more such episodes weekly (American Psychiatric Association, 2022). See Table 2 below for an overview of bulimia nervosa diagnostic criteria.

Beyond severity specifiers, the DSM-5-TR indicates that for a person to be diagnosed with bulimia nervosa, the symptoms above cannot occur exclusively in the context of anorexia nervosa (American Psychiatric Association, 2022). Given that there is a binge-eating purging type of anorexia nervosa, many people question how this type of anorexia nervosa differs from bulimia nervosa, with its pattern of binge-eating followed by inappropriate compensatory behaviors. The key difference is in the degree of body weight and starvation. To be diagnosed with anorexia nervosa, a person must have a significantly low body weight resulting from severe food restriction. On the other hand, a person with bulimia nervosa need not restrict food to be diagnosed. Furthermore, there is no requirement for a person to be fearful of weight gain for bulimia nervosa diagnosis. So, the binge-eating/purging type of anorexia is diagnosed when binging and purging behaviors occur within the overall context of a disorder involving restriction, low body weight, and intense fear of weight gain. In bulimia nervosa, binge-purge behaviors, not restriction, are the central diagnostic feature of the disorder. Another key distinction between the two is that a person must show both binging and purging behaviors to be diagnosed with bulimia nervosa. On the other hand, the binge-eating/purging type of anorexia requires binge-eating or purging behavior, so both behaviors need not be present for diagnosis (American Psychiatric Association, 2022). It is critical to understand these key distinctions for the purpose of making an accurate diagnosis.

Table 2. Bulimia nervosa diagnostic criteria

General Diagnostic Criteria
• Recurrent episodes of binge eating that involve consuming much more food than a typical person would eat under similar circumstances and that involve a sense that one has lost control over how much they're eating • Repeated inappropriate compensatory behaviors, such as excessive exercise, self-induced vomiting, fasting, or laxative misuse, which is undertaken to prevent weight gain from binging and occurs at least once a week for 3 months • Overemphasis on body weight and shape when evaluating oneself • Symptoms that do not occur exclusively in the context of anorexia nervosa
Severity Specifiers
• Mild: 1-3 episodes of inappropriate compensatory behaviors per week, on average • Moderate: 4-7 episodes of inappropriate compensatory behaviors per week, on average • Severe: 8-13 episodes of inappropriate compensatory behaviors per week, on average • Extreme: 14 or more episodes of inappropriate compensatory behaviors per week, on average
Other Specifiers
• In partial remission: After previously meeting all of the general diagnostic criteria noted above, some but not all of the criteria have been met for a sustained period of time. • In full remission: A person previously met full criteria for bulimia nervosa but has not met any of the general diagnostic criteria above for a sustained period.

Binge-Eating Disorder

Binge-eating disorder is a distinct condition from anorexia nervosa and bulimia nervosa, as it does not involve disturbances in body image or overemphasis on weight and shape when evaluating oneself. To be diagnosed with binge eating disorder, a person must engage in recurrent binge-eating episodes, which involve both eating a significantly larger amount of food than the typical person would eat over a given time period, and feeling a lack of control over the amount of food consumed during the binge. A person must meet three of the following five criteria related to binges to be diagnosed: eating much more rapidly than normal when binging, eating to the point of uncomfortable fullness, consuming large quantities of food even when not hungry, eating alone due to embarrassment over the amount consumed, and feeling disgusted, depressed, or guilty following the binge. Other diagnostic criteria include the experience of significant distress related to binges as well as binge eating that occurs at least weekly for three months. Binges cannot occur in the context of bulimia, in which there are inappropriate compensatory behaviors to rid the body of excess calories (American Psychiatric Association, 2022).

As is the case with anorexia and bulimia nervosa, there are severity specifiers for binge-eating disorder. The disorder is considered mild when a person has one to three binge-eating episodes per week, moderate when there are four to seven binges per week, severe when there are eight to 13 binges per week, and extreme when there are 14 or more binge-eating episodes in one week. See Table 3 below for a depiction of the full diagnostic criteria for binge-eating disorder.

Table 3. Binge-eating disorder diagnostic criteria

General Diagnostic Criteria
• Recurrent episodes of binge eating that involve consuming much more food than a typical person would eat under similar circumstances and that involve a sense that one has lost control over how much they're eating • Experiencing at least three of the following symptoms in relation to the binge-eating episodes: eating much faster than normal, eating to the point of being uncomfortably full, eating large amounts of food even when not hungry, eating alone due to embarrassment, or feeling a sense of disgust, depression, or guilt after binging • Binging at least once a week, on average, for 3 months • Binging does not involve recurrent compensatory behaviors, as is the case with bulimia nervosa
Severity Specifiers
• Mild: 1-3 episodes of binging per week, on average • Moderate: 4-7 episodes of binging per week, on average • Severe: 8-13 episodes of binging per week, on average • Extreme: 14 or more episodes of binging per week, on average
Other Specifiers
• In partial remission: After previously meeting all of the general diagnostic criteria noted above, a person has engaged in binge eating less than once per week on average over a sustained period of time. • In full remission: A person previously met full criteria for binge-eating disorder but has not met any of the general diagnostic criteria above for a sustained period.

Pica

Not all eating disorders involve body image disturbances or feeling a loss of control over food intake. In fact, there are several eating disorders that are not linked to these disturbances, and pica is one such disorder. The primary diagnostic feature of pica is the ongoing consumption of non-food substances that have no nutritional value, for a period of a month or more. Other diagnostic criteria include the fact that the eating disturbance cannot be appropriate to the person's developmental level, nor can it be part of a culturally or socially appropriate practice. It can occur alongside another mental health disorder, such as autism spectrum disorder, or a medical condition, like pregnancy, but it must be severe enough that it necessitates its own clinical attention There is just one specifier for pica—in remission—which is utilized when a person previously met diagnostic criteria for pica but has not met criteria for a sustained time (American Psychiatric Association, 2022).

Rumination Disorder

Rumination disorder is another eating disorder that does not involve disturbances related to poor body image or loss of control over eating. The primary feature of this disorder is regurgitating food repeatedly, over a period lasting at least one month. An individual with rumination disorder may spit out regurgitated food, or they may re-chew or re-swallow it. To be diagnosed, regurgitation cannot be due to a medical condition like gastroesophageal reflux, nor can it occur exclusively in the context of anorexia nervosa, bulimia nervosa, binge-eating disorder, or avoidant/restrictive food intake disorder. Symptoms of regurgitation can occur alongside another mental disorder, such as intellectual developmental disorder, but they must be severe enough to necessitate their own clinical attention. Like pica, there is just one specifier for rumination disorder—in remission—which is utilized when a person previously met diagnostic criteria for rumination disorder but has not met criteria for a sustained time (American Psychiatric Association, 2022).

Avoidant/Restrictive Food Intake Disorder

Avoidant/restrictive food intake disorder is also among the feeding and eating disorders, and it does not involve a disturbance in body image. Individuals with avoidant/restrictive food intake disorder show an eating disturbance that involves at least one of these symptoms: significant weight loss or failure to gain weight as expected during childhood; noteworthy nutritional deficiency; reliance on nutrition supplements or enteral feeding; or difficulty with psychosocial functioning arising from the feeding disturbance. Individuals with avoidant/restrictive food intake disorder do not avoid food because of fear of weight gain; instead, the avoidance is based on a lack of interest in eating, displeasure with the sensory experience of eating, or worry that eating will bring about unpleasant side effects. Other diagnostic criteria for the disorder include that it cannot be explained by limited food access or a common cultural practice, nor can it occur only in the context of anorexia or bulimia nervosa. A person cannot show a disturbance in body image, nor can the eating behavior be explained by a medical condition. There is one specifier for avoidant/restrictive food intake disorder—in remission—which is used when a person previously met full criteria for the disorder but has not met the criteria for a sustained time period (American Psychiatric Association, 2022).

Unspecified and Other Specified Feeding or Eating Disorder

Not everyone who struggles with eating-related disturbances will fit nicely into the diagnostic criteria for one of the specific disorders in the DSM-5-TR. Given this fact, the manual contains two disorders that can be utilized for those who experience significant distress or dysfunction related to feeding and eating disturbances, but who do not meet diagnostic criteria for another disorder. The diagnosis of other specified feeding or eating disorder is given to individuals who have symptoms of such a disorder but who do not meet full criteria for another disorder in the chapter on feeding and eating disorders; this diagnosis is given when the clinician specifies the reason a patient does not meet criteria for another feeding and eating disorder (American Psychiatric Association, 2022).

The DSM-5-TR offers several examples of eating disorder presentations that can align with the diagnosis of other specified feeding or eating disorder (American Psychiatric Association, 2022):

- **Atypical anorexia nervosa:** A presentation of anorexia nervosa in which all diagnostic criteria are met, aside from the requirement of being at a significantly low body weight.
- **Bulimia nervosa (of low frequency and limited duration):** A presentation of bulimia in which all diagnostic criteria are met, but binge eating and compensatory behaviors do not occur at least once a week on average and/or for at least 3 months.
- **Binge-eating disorder (of low frequency and/or limited duration):** A presentation of binge-eating disorder in which all diagnostic criteria are met, but binge-eating behaviors do not occur at least once a week on average and/or for at least 3 months.
- **Purging disorder:** A presentation of a feeding and eating disorder in which a person repeatedly purges, such as by forcing vomiting or misusing laxatives, to lose weight, but does not engage in binge eating.
- **Night eating syndrome:** A presentation of a feeding and eating disorder in which a person has repeated episodes of eating during the night after waking up from sleep, or of consuming excessive amounts of food after the evening meal.

The presentations above meet criteria for other specified feeding or eating disorder, as they allow for identifying the specific reason a person does not meet criteria for another disorder in the feeding and eating disorders chapter. An unspecified feeding or eating disorder, on the other hand, is diagnosed when a person does not meet criteria for another disorder in the chapter, and the clinician does not specify the reason the patient does not meet criteria for another disorder. This diagnosis would be appropriate in contexts in which the clinician doesn't have enough information to make another diagnosis, such as when assessing patients in a hospital emergency department (American Psychiatric Association, 2022).

DIAGNOSTIC TOOLS

Diagnosing a feeding and eating disorder requires the clinician to review the diagnostic criteria in the DSM-5-TR, as described in the previous section, to determine if a patient meets criteria for a diagnosis. There are diagnostic tools available to assist clinicians with this process. Knowing where to begin with eating disorder assessment can be challenging, so it can be helpful to utilize a screening tool. The SCOFF, developed by Morgan et al. (1999) has been identified as valid for detecting anorexia and bulimia nervosa in women (Kutz et al., 2020). If either of these disorders is suspected, using the SCOFF can be a suitable starting point for assessment. This tool asks the following five questions:

"Do you make yourself **Sick** *because you feel uncomfortably full?*

Do you worry you have lost **Control** *over how much you eat?*

Have you recently lost more than **One** *stone in a 3 month period?*

Do you believe yourself to be **Fat** *when others say you are too thin?*

Would you say that **Food** *dominates your life?"*

(Morgan et al., 1999).

The SCOFF is scored by assigning one point for every "yes" answer above. A score of two or more indicates a likely diagnosis of anorexia nervosa or bulimia nervosa, which would suggest that the clinician should utilize criteria in the DSM-5-TR to determine if a person meets diagnostic criteria for either disorder (Morgan et al., 1999). When an eating disorder is expected, The Eating Disorder Assessment for DSM-5 (EDA-5) is a useful tool. The EDA-5 has been found to be reliable and valid for diagnosing eating disorders, and it can be used to assess for anorexia nervosa, bulimia nervosa, and binge-eating disorder (Sysko et al., 2015). This electronic assessment tool is available online for no charge, at eda5.org. It asks the following questions (Glasofer et al., 2016):

"Are you having problems with your eating? For example, is it hard for you to maintain your weight or alter your diet? Do other people feel you have a problem in these areas?"

"Can you describe a typical day of eating? When and what do you eat?"

"Is the problem with your eating getting in the way of your day-to-day functioning? For example, at work, at school or in your relationships?"

"Is the problem interfering with your health? Is it very distressing or upsetting to you?"

"What are your current height and weight?"

"What was your lowest weight in the last 3 months?"

"Are you afraid of gaining weight?"

"If no, are you worried that if you start to gain weight, you will continue to gain weight and will become fat?"

"Do you try to cut back on calories or amounts or types of food? What do you try to do?"

"Do you exercise? What do you do and how often?"

"Do you vomit or use any types of pills (such as diet pills diuretics, or laxatives)?"

"Do you do anything else that might make it hard for you to gain or maintain weight?"

"In terms of your body weight and shape, how do you think you look?"

"Does what you see/feel/experience differ from how others might perceive you?"

"Have you recently thought that you are fat or that a part of your body is too big?"

"Have you recently had a distorted view of your body? Can you describe it?"

"Does your body shape or weight impact how you feel about yourself? For example, if you were to have a day when you did not like the number on the scale, or the way your clothes fit, or how your body shape felt in general, how much would that impact you? Would it make you feel very badly about yourself? Please tell me a little about this."

"Do you think that your current or recent low weight presents a significant problem for you and your overall health? Why or why not? If yes, what efforts have you made in the last 3 months to deal with this problem? Have your feelings about the significance of the problem fluctuated? How so?"

"In the past 3 months, were there times when you felt a sense of loss of control over eating? Or times when you felt that you could not stop eating? Or times when you felt unable to control what or how much you were eating? If no, have there been times when you felt you could not prevent yourself from eating?"

"Do you make yourself vomit, or overuse (misuse) laxatives, diuretics, or other medications?"

"Do you exercise? What type of exercise do you do and for how long? Does the amount of exercise you do interfere with your health or get in the way of daily responsibilities?"

"Have you eaten any non-food materials (e.g., dirt, paint) in the last month? What have you eaten? How often?"

The assessment above is completed entirely online, with the clinician asking questions of the patient and then selecting whether the patient meets the diagnostic criterion addressed by the question. At the end of the assessment, a diagnosis will be given, based on responses.

Other Quality Diagnostic Tools

The advantage of the EDA-5 is that it can be completed online, and it yields a diagnosis at the end of the assessment, making it a time-efficient method for assessing and diagnosing eating disorders. However, this is not the only diagnostic tool available. Another diagnostic tool, which is considered by many to be the gold standard for eating disorder assessment, is the Eating Disorder Examination (EDE). The EDE has been utilized for decades, and it is based on diagnostic criteria from the 4th edition of the *Diagnostic and Statistical Manual of Mental Disorders.* The EDE has been found to be both reliable and valid; however, it is lacking items relevant to the diagnosis of pica, rumination disorder, and avoidant/restrictive food intake disorder. The EDE is available online free of charge, but compared to the EDA-5, it is more time-consuming to complete and requires significant training (Tournayre et al., 2024).

An alternative to the EDE, the Eating Pathology Symptom Inventory – Clinician-rated version (EPSI-CRV), requires less time to administer. The EPSI-CRV has shown acceptable reliability and validity, and it also includes a self-report form. The EPSI-CRV is able to generate a diagnosis based on the DSM-5, and it assesses cognitive, behavioral, attitudinal, and perceptual dimensions of eating disorders (Tournayre et al., 2024). Like many other eating disorder diagnostic tools, the EPSI-CRV is available online at no charge. The University of Kansas Center for the Advancement of Research on Eating Behaviors provides copies of the EPSI-CRV, as well as the self-report version. The assessment is available in alternative languages, including German and Chinese. The University of Kansas also provides instructions for administration at https://care.ku.edu/epsi.

While there are numerous assessment tools that can be useful for diagnosing eating disorders, many of them are more suitable for diagnosing anorexia nervosa, bulimia nervosa, and binge-eating disorder. The tools described above may not be as reliable and valid for diagnosing pica, rumination disorder, and avoidant/restrictive food intake disorder. In cases in which one of these three disorders is suspected, the Eating Disorders in Youth-Questionnaire may be more appropriate. This assessment tool primarily assesses for symptoms of avoidant/restrictive food intake disorder, with items such as, "I am a picky eater" and "Food/eating does not interest me." There is also one item each that assesses for pica and rumination disorder, respectively (Hilbert & van Dyck, 2016). While this assessment tool was developed primarily to assess for eating disorder symptoms in children, it has been successfully utilized to identify avoidant/restrictive food intake disorder in adults (Hilbert et al., 2021).

CONCLUDING REMARKS

The DSM-5-TR outlines diagnostic criteria for feeding and eating disorders, and clinicians use these criteria in practice to diagnose eating disorders. While two eating disorders, anorexia nervosa and bulimia nervosa, involve a self-image that is unduly based upon body shape and weight, not all disorders in this chapter involve disturbances or obsession with body image. In fact, binge-eating disorder involves episodes of binge-eating, without compensatory behaviors or any fixation on body image. Furthermore, pica, rumination disorder, and avoidant/restrictive food intake disorder involve disturbances in eating that are not accompanied by fixation on body shape or a desire to lose weight (American Psychiatric Association, 2022). When diagnosing eating disorders, it is essential for clinicians to remember that these disorders involve more than just restricting calories or purging excess calories in order to change weight or body shape. The chapter on feeding and eating disorders includes a diverse range of disorders, each of which involves disturbances in eating behaviors. Given the diverse range of eating disorders, it can be helpful to use diagnostic tools to assist with arriving at a diagnosis.

REFERENCES

American Psychiatric Association. (2022). *Diagnostic and statistical manual of mental disorders* (5th ed., text rev.)., DOI: 10.1176/appi.books.9780890425787

Glasofer, D. R., Sysko, R., & Walsh, B. T. (2016). The use of the Eating Disorder Assessment for DSM-5 (EDA-5). In Sysko, R., Glasofer, D. R., Attia, E., & Walsh, B. T. (Eds.), *Handbook of Assessment and Treatment of Eating Disorders* (pp. 175–206). American Psychiatric Association.

Guarda, A. (2023). *What are eating disorders?* American Psychiatric Association. https://www.psychiatry.org/patients-families/eating-disorders/what-are-eating-disorders

Hilbert, A., & van Dyck, Z. (2016). *Eating Disorders in Youth-Questionnaire. English version.* University of Leipzig: http://nbn-resolving.de/urn:nbn:de:bsz:15-qucosa-197246

Hilbert, A., Zenger, M., Eichler, J., & Brähler, E. (2021). Psychometric evaluation of the Eating Disorders in Youth-Questionnaire when used in adults: Prevalence estimates for symptoms of avoidant/restrictive food intake disorder and population norms. *International Journal of Eating Disorders*, *54*(3), 399–408. DOI: 10.1002/eat.23424 PMID: 33283329

Kutz, A. M., Marsh, A. G., Gunderson, C. G., Maguen, S., & Masheb, R. M. (2020). Eating disorder screening: A systematic review and meta-analysis of diagnostic test characteristics of the SCOFF. *Journal of General Internal Medicine*, *35*(3), 885–893. DOI: 10.1007/s11606-019-05478-6 PMID: 31705473

Morgan, J. F., Reid, F., & Lacey, J. H. (1999). The SCOFF questionnaire: Assessment of a new screening tool for eating disorders. *BMJ (Clinical Research Ed.)*, *319*(7223), 1467–1468. DOI: 10.1136/bmj.319.7223.1467 PMID: 10582927

Sysko, R., Glasofer, D. R., Hildebrandt, T., Klimek, P., Mitchell, J. E., Berg, K. C., Peterson, C. B., Wonderlich, S. A., & Walsh, B. T. (2015). The eating disorder assessment for DSM-5 (EDA-5): Development and validation of a structured interview for feeding and eating disorders. *International Journal of Eating Disorders*, *48*(5), 452–463. DOI: 10.1002/eat.22388 PMID: 25639562

Tournayre, L., Balbinotti, M. A. A., & Monthuy-Blanc, J. (2024). Some hope for a dimensional assessment? A critical review of psychometric validated (semi-)structured interview to assess eating disorders. *European Eating Disorders Review*, *32*(6), 1138–1156. DOI: 10.1002/erv.3115 PMID: 38873932

KEY TERMS AND DEFINITIONS

Anorexia Nervosa: An eating disorder characterized by food restriction, low body weight, extreme fear of weight gain, and body image disturbance or fixation.

Avoidant/Restrictive Food Intake Disorder: An eating disorder in which a person avoids food due to anxiety, displeasure with food, or lack of desire to eat.

Binge-Eating Disorder: An eating disorder involving repeat episodes of binging, during which a person loses control over food consumption and then experiences side effects like disgust, depression, or preferring to eat alone because of binge-eating.

Bulimia Nervosa: An eating disorder in which a person who is fixated on body weight and shape repeatedly engages in binge-eating and then uses inappropriate compensatory behaviors like laxative misuse or self-induced vomiting to compensate for binges.

Other Specified Feeding or Eating Disorder: A diagnosis given when a person shows eating disorder symptoms but does not meet full criteria for a specific eating disorder in this chapter, and the clinician specifies why a person cannot be diagnosed with another specific eating disorder.

Pica: An eating disorder involving the consumption of non-food material that offers no nutritional value.

Rumination Disorder: An eating disorder characterized by repeated regurgitation of food.

Unspecified Feeding or Eating Disorder: A diagnosis given when a person shows eating disorder symptoms but does not meet full criteria for a specific eating disorder in this chapter, and the clinician does not specify why a person cannot be diagnosed with another specific disorder.

Chapter 2
Eating Disorder Risk Factors and Epidemiology

ABSTRACT

This chapter explores the complex risk factors associated with feeding and eating disorders, emphasizing the interplay of family-related, individual, genetic, and cultural influences in their development. The chapter begins by discussing the diversity of eating disorders, including anorexia nervosa, bulimia nervosa, binge eating disorder (BED), avoidant/restrictive food intake disorder (ARFID), rumination disorder, and pica. Given the distinct characteristics of each disorder, risk factors are examined separately, with special attention to how they differ across diagnostic categories. The chapter concludes with a discussion of the prevalence of the various eating disorders.

BACKGROUND

As discussed in the previous chapter, there is not one singular presentation of an eating disorder; instead, there are a variety of different disorders that fall under the umbrella of a feeding and eating disorder (American Psychiatric Association, 2022). Just as there are a variety of different eating disorders, there are a range of risk factors that can contribute to eating disorder development. These risk factors can also vary, based upon

DOI: 10.4018/979-8-3373-0664-3.ch002

the type of eating disorder. This chapter seeks to describe the various risk factors for eating disorders, with these risk factors separated by the specific eating disorder type. For instance, risk factors for anorexia nervosa are presented differently from risk factors for bulimia nervosa. The chapter concludes with a section on epidemiology, discussing the prevalence of various eating disorders within the population.

RISK FACTORS FOR ANOREXIA NERVOSA

Numerous risk factors contribute to the development of anorexia nervosa. Among these risk factors, the contribution of family-related factors has been well-researched. Del Casale et al. (2023) conducted a systematic review of familial risk factors for anorexia nervosa (AN) and concluded, "The onset and maintenance of AN seems to be closely related to familial risk factors, and knowing them is crucial to identify the best therapeutic approach in order to target the unhealthy family environment as well as the needs of the patient" (p. 25478). The identified familial risk factors for anorexia nervosa are numerous and include relational trauma, history of psychiatric disorders in the family, expectations of perfectionism within the family, overall family dysfunction, family conflict, emotional reactivity in the family, low levels of family involvement, negative emotions within the family, taboos related to sexuality and nudity, and the loss of an important family member during the mother's pregnancy (Del Casale et al., 2023).

The findings of Del Casale et al. (2023) agree with earlier research which has found that family risk factors, including having a sibling with anorexia nervosa and having a history of mood disorders in the family, are predictive of the development of anorexia nervosa (Steinhausen et al., 2015). Hilbert et al. (2014) arrived at similar conclusions, finding that problem parenting, family dieting and overeating, parental substance use disorder, demanding parenting, and parental mood were all linked to the development of anorexia nervosa. Beyond general family risk factors, mothers have been found to play an influential role in the development of behaviors related to anorexia nervosa. For example, Haynos et al. (2016) found that maternal dieting was linked to a risk of escalating restrictive eating behaviors in children, as are seen in anorexia nervosa. These researchers also found that poor family communication increased the risk of restrictive eating behaviors, adding additional support for the strong link between family-related risk factors and anorexia nervosa (Haynos et al., 2016). While some familial risk factors linked to anorexia nervosa may occur because of environmental concerns, such as poor communication or modeling of unhealthy eating behaviors, genetics also play a central role in family-related risk. People who have a relative with anorexia nervosa are 11 times more likely to develop the disorder when compared to those without a family history, suggesting a strong genetic component (Barakat et al., 2023).

Interestingly, family-related factors appear to be linked to anorexia nervosa risk across cultures. A Portuguese study revealed that parents' history of eating disorders, as well as critical comments concerning weight, shape, or food consumption, were predictors of anorexia nervosa (Machado et al., 2014). A Japanese study also found that family-related factors increased the risk of anorexia nervosa, with family relationship problems and parental mental health issues being linked to the development of this disorder. There were some nuanced differences in anorexia risk factors in Japan compare to the United States, but the fact remains that family risk factors are seen in diverse cultural contexts (Pike et al., 2021).

There is extensive evidence that risk factors within the family can lead to the development of anorexia nervosa, but there are additional factors that contribute to this eating disorder. For example, individual risk factors also contribute, with low-self esteem and depressive symptoms predicting the onset of restrictive eating behaviors (Haynos et al., 2016). Other individual factors, including dissatisfaction with one's body during childhood, are also linked to the development of anorexia nervosa, especially for girls (Micali et al., 2015). In addition, having a perfectionistic personality is a risk factor for anorexia nervosa, and this personality trait can actually separate those at risk of anorexia from those at risk of other eating disorders, including binge-eating disorder (Hilbert et al., 2014). Additional research has confirmed that individual psychosocial characteristics increase the risk of anorexia nervosa. Compared to healthy controls, those with anorexia nervosa show higher levels of psychological maladjustment, experiencing more interpersonal and emotional problems, as well as lower self-esteem, higher desire to be thin, greater body dissatisfaction, higher levels of emotional emptiness, increased emotional dysregulation, and higher insecurity in interpersonal relationships (Batista et al., 2018). Additionally, Batista et al. (2018) found that those with anorexia nervosa presented with high levels of perfectionism, and they utilized self-denial and suffering to pursue perfection.

There are other individual risk factors that can predict the onset of anorexia nervosa. For instance, dieting has consistently been associated with the onset of anorexia nervosa (Hilbert et al., 2014; Stice et al., 2017). Finally, individuals with anorexia nervosa are likely to demonstrate negative affect and impairment in daily functioning, making these traits risks factors for the eating disorder (Stice et al., 2017).

Both individual and family risk factors contribute to the development of anorexia nervosa, but a discussion of risk factors for this eating disorder would be incomplete without addressing macro-level factors, such as the influence of culture and mass media. Izydorczyk et al. (2020) found that sociocultural pressures related to thinness were linked to restrictive eating in women, suggesting that these pressures could be a risk factor for anorexia nervosa. Shaefer et al. (2019) found that even moderate internalization of the thin ideal was associated with pathological eating behaviors, showing just how powerful cultural ideals can be in the development of eating disorders like anorexia nervosa. Closely related to cultural values is the impact of peer relationships, which can influence dieting behavior and increase body dissatisfaction, thereby increasing eating disorder risk (Quiles Marcos et al., 2013). Finally, social media use can increase the risk of anorexia nervosa via social comparison and exposure to the thin ideal (Dane & Bhatia, 2023).

Beyond factors within the larger cultural landscape, it appears that factors related to one's racial and ethnic background can contribute to anorexia nervosa risk. For example, research has found that those who identify as biracial have higher risk of anorexia nervosa when compared to other racial and ethnic groups, which can be related to the cultural experience of navigating multiple identities and coping with discrimination. In addition, indigenous populations have a higher risk of anorexia than other groups. They are over twice as likely to be diagnosed with anorexia as Whites, and nearly four times as likely as Blacks to receive an anorexia diagnosis. Intergenerational trauma and acculturation from European colonization have been offered as explanations of the higher anorexia nervosa risk in indigenous groups, as these experiences can contribute to disordered eating and unsafe weight loss practices (Van Dyne at al., 2023).

In summary, a multitude of risk factors contributes to the development of anorexia nervosa. Family-related risk factors play a central role in the development of this eating disorder (Del Casale et al., 2023), but cultural ideals related to thinness can also exert an influence and elevate the risk of anorexia nervosa (Izydorczyk et al., 2020; Schaefer et al., 2019). Similarly, peer and social media influences can also affect eating behaviors and internalization of thin ideals, thereby increasing the risk for anorexia nervosa (Dane & Bhatia, 2023; Quiles Marcos et al., 2013). The experiences associated with membership in a particular ethnic or racial group can also increase the risk of anorexia nervosa (Van Dyne at al., 2023). While family and culture-related influences contribute strongly to anorexia nervosa risk, individual risk factors also play a role. Individual factors, including psychological maladjustment, perfectionism, negative affect, dieting behavior, depression, and body dissatisfaction are also linked to anorexia nervosa (Batista et al., 2018; Haynos et al., 2016; Hilbert et al., 2014; Micali et al., 2015; Stice et al., 2017). Based on the body of research on risk factors for anorexia nervosa, the most reasonable conclusion is that there is not one single factor that causes this eating disorder. Rather, in any individual case of anorexia nervosa, a combination of risk factors likely contributes to the development of the disorder.

RISK FACTORS FOR BULIMIA NERVOSA

Bulimia nervosa is a distinct condition with separate diagnostic features from anorexia nervosa. As such, it is necessary to describe bulimia nervosa risk factors separately. As is the case with anorexia, family-related risk factors for bulimia nervosa are present. For instance, having low parental support has been identified as a risk factor for bulimia (Yamamiya & Stice, 2024). Trauma is another risk factor that can occur in the context of the family environment and increase the risk of bulimia nervosa. Various forms of trauma are linked to eating disorders, and trauma specifically increases the risk of bulimia nervosa. For women, trauma from emotional abuse is linked to the development of eating disorders, whereas for men, trauma from physical or sexual abuse increases eating disorder risk. Having a history of multiple types of child maltreatment increases the risk of bulimia-related behaviors like purging. Similarly, family disruption, such as that which occurs with divorce, separation, or removal from the parental home, increases bulimia nervosa risk (Barakat et al., 2023; Hilbert et al., 2014).

Other family-related risk factors for bulimia include poor parenting skills in both parents, family conflict, and growing up with demanding parents. Family eating behaviors, which include both dieting behavior and overeating, are also linked to increased risk of bulimia nervosa. Finally, a family history of bulimia nervosa also increases the risk that a person will develop this disorder (Hilbert et al., 2014). It is possible that genetic factors play a role in the relationship between family history and bulimia risk, with different studies showing that the heritability of the disorder rangers from 28%-83% (Donato et al., 2022).

Family risk factors are not the only contributors to bulimia nervosa risk, as personal characteristics also play a role. For instance, bulimia risk is higher in those who have a history of conduct problems, as well as in those with a history of childhood obesity. Similar to anorexia nervosa, perfectionism and negative emotionality also elevate the risk of bulimia nervosa (Hilbert et al., 2014). Other individual risk factors associated with increased risk of bulimia nervosa include internalization of thin ideals, experiencing pressure to be thin, and being dissatisfied with one's body ((Yamamiya & Stice, 2024).

Having another psychiatric disorder, such as depression or anxiety, may also be an individual risk factor for bulimia nervosa. Numerous studies have shown that depression and anxiety are significantly more common in those with bulimia nervosa when compared to healthy controls. One proposed mechanism for this relationship is the mediating role of low self-esteem in depression and anxiety, which can lead to body dissatisfaction and thus disordered eating behaviors (Zanella & Lee, 2022). As Zanella and Lee (2022) have stated, "Depression and anxiety are potent risk factors for the development of problematic eating."

Two other important individual factors linked to bulimia are attachment-related anxiety and emotion regulation difficulties. Individuals with bulimia nervosa demonstrate higher levels of emotion regulation difficulties compared to healthy controls. Furthermore, attachment-related anxiety predicts bulimia nervosa symptoms, which establishes insecure attachment as a potential risk factor for the disorder (Jakovina et al., 2018).

Individual traits including attachment anxiety can contribute to bulimia risk, and as is the case with anorexia nervosa, cultural factors also seem to play a role in risk. Some research suggests that the highest prevalence of bulimia nervosa exists in Whites, with the lowest rates in African Americans, a difference which is statistically significant. This suggests cultural factors may play some role in the risk for bulimia (Ruchkin et al., 2021). Other research has found relatively similar levels of eating disorders, including bulimia, among White, Hispanic American, African American, and Asian American women. However, Asian American women were found to have higher internalization of the thin ideal when compared to both White and African American women. Furthermore, Whites had a higher level of internalization of the thin ideal than African American women, which could be a cultural factor that explains, at least in part, the higher rates of bulimia nervosa in Whites (Cheng et al., 2019). Still further research has found that indigenous individuals are more likely than any other race to experience a bulimia nervosa diagnosis; they are almost three times as likely as Blacks to have a bulimia diagnosis and just over two times as likely as Whites to have such a diagnosis. Researchers have theorized that indigenous populations may be at increased risk of bulimia due to acculturation and intergenerational trauma from European colonization. In addition, those who identify as biracial are at higher risk of bulimia nervosa than other races, which researchers have attributed to experiences of oppression and the difficulty that comes with navigating multiple identities (Van Dyne et al., 2023). Regardless of the exact mechanisms by which it occurs, increased risk of bulimia nervosa among certain racial/ethnic groups suggests that cultural risk factors can play a role in the development of this eating disorder.

Beyond factors related to racial and ethnic background, larger cultural norms can contribute to bulimia nervosa risk. More specifically, the mass media, which communicates cultural standards related to body image and appearance, can play a role in bulimic behaviors. The role of cultural expectations communicated in the media tends to differ for men compared to women. For instance, men seem to be more likely to internalize cultural norms related to physical appearance when encountering these norms in the media. On the other hand, women may turn to the media as a source of information about body standards, which increases their risk of bulimia (Izydorczyk et al., 2020).

In conclusion, a variety of risk factors contributes to the development of bulimia nervosa. Family risk factors, including trauma and abuse occurring within the family, can increase the risk of bulimia nervosa (Barakat et al., 2023; Hilbert et al., 2014; Yamamiya & Stice, 2024). Some of the family-related risk for bulimia nervosa may be the result of genetic factors (Donato et al., 2022). Individual risk factors also contribute to bulimia nervosa risk. Such risk factors include conduct problems, childhood obesity, perfectionism, tendency toward negative emotionality, internalization of thin ideals, feeling pressure to be thin, experiencing body dissatisfaction, difficulties with emotion regulation, and attachment anxiety (Hilbert et al., 2014; Jakovina et al., 2022; Yamamiya & Stice, 2024; Zanella & Lee, 2022). Finally, macro-level factors, related to both race and ethnicity and cultural norms pertaining to body image, can contribute to the risk for bulimia nervosa (Cheng et al., 2019; Izydorczyk et al., 2020; Ruchkin et al., 2021; Van Dyne et al., 2023).

RISK FACTORS FOR BINGE-EATING DISORDER

Research indicates that binge-eating disorder (BED) is influenced by a combination of genetic, psychological, and environmental factors. First, as is seen with both anorexia and bulimia, family-related factors contribute to the risk of BED. For example, being separated from a parent, having a family history of bulimia nervosa, and experiencing parental absence or death are all linked to BED risk. Furthermore, family overeating is predictive of binge eating disorder. Trauma occurring within the family context, such as experiencing sexual abuse, can also increase the risk of BED (Hilbert et al., 2014).

As noted above, family-related risk factors such as overeating and parental absence can increase the risk of BED, but some of the risk within families is genetic. Twin studies show that the genetic contribution to BED ranges from 39% to 45%, suggesting that genetic factors play a moderate role in the development of this eating disorder (Steiger & Booij, 2020). Genetic research further suggests that BED is a specific type of obesity associated with being particularly sensitive to the rewarding, pleasurable aspects of food. This sensitivity to reward can be affected by two specific genes, Taq1A and A118G, which influence the functioning of the brain's reward system. Some research also suggests that genes linked to the serotonin system can increase BED risk (Davis, 2015).

Beyond family and genetic risk factors, individual characteristics may increase the risk of binge eating disorder. First, personality traits like high anxiety and a tendency toward impulsivity are linked to a higher risk of BED (Davis, 2015). Psychologically, individuals with BED often experience body dissatisfaction, internalization of the thin ideal, and higher rates of substance abuse than those without BED. Other individual factors linked to BED risk include history of pregnancy, conduct problems, severe childhood obesity, and being bullied or teased. Furthermore, as is the case with both anorexia and bulimia, negative emotionality is associated with a higher risk of binge eating (Hilbert et al., 2014; Stice at al., 2017).

Mental health problems may also be predictive of BED. Research has revealed that up to 94% of those with BED have experienced mental health symptoms during their lifetimes. Mood disorders, substance use disorders, and anxiety disorders are highly prevalent in those with BED. While less common than the aforementioned, PTSD and borderline personality disorder are also common in those with BED (Keski-Rahkonen, 2021). Given that seeking mental health care is predictive for the development of BED, it is reasonable to conclude that mental health disorders can precede BED and thus be risk factors for the later development of this eating disorder (Stice et al., 2017).

Finally, it's important to consider cultural factors that may contribute to BED development. Rodgers et al. (2018) have found that BED tends to be most common in Latino populations. Furthermore, these researchers discovered that the course of BED tends to differ for Hispanic and Latino populations when compared to Black and White groups. The former tends to first begin with binge eating and then move on to dieting behavior, whereas Blacks and Whites are more likely to begin with dieting and then later progress to binge eating. Furthermore, Latinos have been found to be more fearful of weight gain from binging when compared to Whites, and overeating tends to be more common in Latino populations (Rodgers et al., 2018). This suggests that cultural factors within Hispanic/Latino populations may predispose to binge eating and thus BED.

RISK FACTORS FOR PICA, RUMINATION DISORDER, AND AVOIDANT/RESTRICTIVE FOOD INTAKE DISORDER

This final section on risk factors groups pica, rumination disorder, and avoidant/restrictive food intake disorder together. This is not to suggest that any one of these disorders is any less serious than the others in this section. Rather, these eating disorders have been categorized together, as there is less research available on the factors that contribute to their development.

Pica, rumination disorder, and avoidant/restrictive food intake disorder (ARFID) all have complex etiologies involving family-related, individual, and cultural risk factors. Family dynamics are believed to play a significant role in the development of these disorders. For instance, in ARFID, parental pressure to eat can negatively impact a child's food intake, leading to picky eating and weight issues during childhood. This pressure may disrupt the child's natural hunger cues and also lead to more fussiness around eating (Jansen et al., 2017). Furthermore, parental pressure and ARFID are likely to overlap in children with autism spectrum disorder (Kozak et al., 2023). Additional research suggests that negative, conflictual interactions between mother and child, as well as dysfunctional eating attitudes and mental illness in the mother, can lead to the food aversion seen in conditions like ARFID (Lucarelli et al., 2018). Finally, genetics contribute significantly to the development of ARFID .

In the case of pica and rumination disorder, limited research exists on specific family-related risk factors. However, it is recognized that these disorders often co-occur with other mental health conditions associated with impaired functioning, such as intellectual disabilities and autism spectrum disorder, which can be influenced by family environments. There is some evidence that pica might be more likely in individuals who have a history of trauma, neglect, separation from parents, or a lack of positive interactions with parents. For individuals with rumination disorder, stressful life circumstances, neglect, lack of stimulation, and relationship problems with parents may serve as risk factors. Some research suggests rumination disorder can run in families, but there is a lack of research related to genetic contributors to the disorder (Hartmann, 2015).

Individual characteristics significantly contribute to the risk of developing the disorders noted herein. For ARFID, gastrointestinal problems, food allergies, and a history of vomiting or choking with food are risk factors for the development of the disorder. Generalized anxiety and sensory aversions to food are also risk factors for ARFID (Zimmerman & Fisher, 2017). There is also a high co-occurrence of ARFID and autism spectrum disorder, with research showing that 16.27% of those with ARFID have autism spectrum disorder (Sader et al., 2025). Pica, on the other hand, is often associated with iron-deficiency anemia, malnutrition, and pregnancy (Fawcett et al., 2016; Miao et al., 2015). It also frequently occurs alongside mental health disorders that impair functioning, such as intellectual disabilities and autism spectrum disorder (Fields et al., 2021). There is very little research available related to individual risk factors for rumination disorder, but the available body of knowledge suggests that anxiety depression, and female gender are predictive of rumination disorder (Haworth at al., 2024).

Finally, cultural influences can also play a role in the development of the disorders discussed in this section. More specifically, societal norms and cultural practices can impact eating behaviors and perceptions of food. For example, certain cultural practices may involve the consumption of non-food substances, which could be related to pica behaviors (Placek, 2017). There is a paucity of research available on the cultural influences that can contribute to rumination disorder and ARFID.

PREVALENCE OF EATING DISORDERS

When assessing and treating patients who present with potential eating disorders, it's helpful to understand how prevalent these disorders are. This discussion concludes the current chapter with an overview of the prevalence of the different feeding and eating disorders. Different studies reveal different prevalence estimates, but a recent meta-analysis provides insight into the overall epidemiology of eating disorders across multiple studies. According to this meta-analysis, 1.69% of people have an eating disorder during their lifetimes, and 0.72% have an eating disorder over the year prior to data collection. Broken down into individual eating disorders, 0.16% of people have anorexia during their lifetimes; 0.63% have bulimia, and 1.53% have binge eating disorder. Women may have higher rates of eating disorders, with a lifetime prevalence of 2.58% according to meta-analysis (Qian et al. 2022).

Meta analytic data on the prevalence of ARFID is also available, and the research suggests that the prevalence of this disorder ranges from a conservative estimate of 4.51% to a higher rate of 11.14% (Nicholls-Clow, 2024). Prevalence estimates of rumination disorder show that 0.4% of children and 3.7% of adults experience this eating disorder (Haworth et al., 2024). Finally, research shows that the prevalence of pica in the general population of children is around 3.5%, compared to 23.2% in children with autism spectrum disorder and 28.1% in those with autism spectrum disorder and intellectual disability (Fields et al., 2021). Research with adults has revealed a prevalence of 4.0% in those seeking treatment at weight loss clinics and up to 68% in pregnant women (Miao et al., 2015).

CONCLUDING REMARKS

In conclusion, the development of feeding and eating disorders is influenced by a complex interplay of familial, individual, genetic, and cultural risk factors, with each disorder exhibiting unique yet overlapping risk profiles. Family-related factors, such as parental modeling of disordered eating, critical comments about weight, and trauma, play a significant role in disorders like anorexia nervosa, bulimia nervosa, and binge eating disorder. Genetic predispositions further contribute to eating disorder risk, particularly in cases of anorexia and BED, where heritability estimates suggest a moderate to strong genetic influence. Individual psychological traits, including perfectionism, body dissatisfaction, emotional dysregulation, and negative affect, are common across eating disorders, often interacting with sociocultural influences such as media exposure and internalization of the thin ideal. Additionally, unique risk factors such as autism spectrum disorder, sensory aversions, and gastrointestinal distress are particularly relevant in the development of ARFID, while iron deficiency and nutritional deficiencies are closely linked to pica. Cultural factors further shape eating disorder risk, with differences in prevalence across racial and ethnic groups, often influenced by historical trauma, acculturation, and societal beauty standards. Ultimately, eating disorders arise from a convergence of biological, psychological, and environmental factors, underscoring the need for a multifaceted approach to prevention, assessment, and intervention.

REFERENCES

American Psychiatric Association. (2022). *Diagnostic and statistical manual of mental disorders* (5th ed., text rev.)., DOI: 10.1176/appi.books.9780890425787

Barakat, S., McLean, S. A., Bryant, E., Le, E., Marks, P., Touyz, S., & Maguire, S. (2023). Risk factors for eating disorders: Findings from a rapid review. *Journal of Eating Disorders*, *11*(8), 1–31. DOI: 10.1186/s40337-022-00717-4 PMID: 36650572

Batista, M., Žigić Antić, L., Žaja, O., Jakovina, T., & Begovac, I. (2018). Predictors of eating disorder risk in anorexia nervosa adolescents. *Acta Clinica Croatica*, *57*(3), 399–410. DOI: 10.20471/acc.2018.57.03.01 PMID: 31168171

Cheng, Z. H., Perko, V. L., Fuller-Marashi, L., Gau, J. M., & Stice, E. (2019). Ethnic differences in eating disorder prevalence, risk factors, and predictive effects of risk factors among young women. *Eating Behaviors*, *32*, 23–30. DOI: 10.1016/j.eatbeh.2018.11.004 PMID: 30529736

Dane, A., & Bhatia, K. (2023). The social media diet: A scoping review to investigate the association between social media, body image, and eating disorders amongst young people. *PLOS Global Public Health*, *3*(3), e0001091. DOI: 10.1371/journal.pgph.0001091 PMID: 36962983

Davis, C. (2015). The epidemiology and genetics of binge eating disorder (BED). *CNS Spectrums*, *20*(6), 522–529. DOI: 10.1017/S1092852915000462 PMID: 26258270

Del Casale, A., Adriani, B., Modesti, M. N., Virzi, S., Parmigiani, G., Vento, A. E., & Speranza, A. M. (2023). Anorexia nervosa and familial risk factors: A systematic review of the literature. *Current Psychology (New Brunswick, N.J.)*, *42*(29), 25476–25484. DOI: 10.1007/s12144-022-03563-4

Donato, K., Ceccarini, M. R., Dhuli, K., Bonetti, G., Medori, M. C., Marceddu, G., Precone, V., Xhufi, S., Bushati, M., Bozo, D., Beccari, T., & Bertelli, M. (2022). Gene variants in eating disorders: Focus on anorexia nervosa, bulimia nervosa, and binge-eating disorder. *Journal of Preventive Medicine and Hygiene*, *63*(2, Suppl 3), E297–E305. DOI: 10.15167/2421-4248/jpmh2022.63.2S3.2772 PMID: 36479493

Fawcett, E. J., Fawcett, J. M., & Mazmanian, D. (2016). A meta-analysis of the worldwide prevalence of pica during pregnancy and the postpartum period. *International Journal of Gynaecology and Obstetrics: the Official Organ of the International Federation of Gynaecology and Obstetrics*, *133*(3), 277–283. DOI: 10.1016/j.ijgo.2015.10.012 PMID: 26892693

Fields, V. L., Soke, G. N., Reynolds, A., Tian, L. H., Wiggins, L., Maenner, M., DiGuiseppi, C., Kral, T. V. E., Hightshoe, K., & Schieve, L. A. (2021). Pica, autism, and other disabilities. *Pediatrics*, *147*(2), e20200462. DOI: 10.1542/peds.2020-0462 PMID: 33408069

Hartmann, A. S. (2015). Pica and rumination disorder. In *Encyclopedia of Feeding and Eating Disorders* (pp. 1–5). Springer., DOI: 10.1007/978-981-287-087-2_40-1

Haworth, J. J., Treadway, S., & Hobson, A. R. (2024). The prevalence of rumination syndrome and rumination disorder: A systematic review and meta-analysis. *Neurogastroenterology and Motility*, *36*(7), e14793. DOI: 10.1111/nmo.14793 PMID: 38563201

Haynos, A. F., Watts, A. W., Loth, K. A., Pearson, C. M., & Neumark-Stzainer, D. (2016). Factors predicting an escalation of restrictive eating during adolescence. *The Journal of Adolescent Health*, *59*(4), 391–396. DOI: 10.1016/j.jadohealth.2016.03.011 PMID: 27161416

Hilbert, A., Pike, K. M., Goldschmidt, A. B., Wilfley, D. E., Fairburn, C. G., Dohm, F. A., Walsh, T., & Striegel Weissman, R. (2014). Risk factors across the eating disorders. *Psychiatry Research*, *220*(1-2), 500–506. DOI: 10.1016/j.psychres.2014.05.054 PMID: 25103674

Izydorczyk, B., Sitnik-Warchulska, K., Lizińczyk, S., & Lipowska, M. (2020). Socio-cultural standards promoted by the mass media as predictors of restrictive and bulimic behavior. *Frontiers in Psychiatry*, *11*, 506. DOI: 10.3389/fpsyt.2020.00506 PMID: 32581880

Jakovina, T., Crnković Batista, M., Ražić Pavičić, A., Žurić Jakovina, I., & Begovac, I. (2018). Emotional dysregulation and attachment dimensions in female patients with bulimia nervosa. *Psychiatria Danubina*, *30*(1), 72–78. DOI: 10.24869/psyd.2018.72 PMID: 29546861

Jansen, P. W., de Barse, L. M., Jaddoe, V. W. V., Verhulst, F. C., Franco, O. H., & Tiemeier, H. (2017). Bi-directional associations between child fussy eating and parents' pressure to eat: Who influences whom? *Physiology & Behavior*, *176*, 101–106. DOI: 10.1016/j.physbeh.2017.02.015 PMID: 28215424

Keski-Rahkonen, A. (2021). Epidemiology of binge eating disorder: Prevalence, course, comorbidity, and risk factors. *Current Opinion in Psychiatry*, *34*(6), 525–531. DOI: 10.1097/YCO.0000000000000750 PMID: 34494972

Kozak, A., Czepczor-Bernat, K., Modrzejewska, J., Modrzejewska, A., Matusik, E., & Matusik, P. (2023). Avoidant/Restrictive Food Disorder (ARFID), food neophobia, other eating-related behaviours and feeding practices among children with autism spectrum disorder and in non-clinical sample: A preliminary study. *International Journal of Environmental Research and Public Health*, *20*(10), 5822. DOI: 10.3390/ijerph20105822 PMID: 37239549

Lucarelli, L., Sechi, C., Cimino, S., & Chatoor, I. (2018). Avoidant/Restrictive Food Intake Disorder: A longitudinal study of malnutrition and psychopathological risk factors from 2 to 11 years of age. *Frontiers in Psychology*, *9*, 1608. DOI: 10.3389/fpsyg.2018.01608 PMID: 30233458

Machado, B. C., Gonçalves, S. F., Martins, C., Hoek, H. W., & Machado, P. P. (2014). Risk factors and antecedent life events in the development of anorexia nervosa: A Portuguese case-control study. *European Eating Disorders Review*, *22*(4), 243–251. DOI: 10.1002/erv.2286 PMID: 24577737

Miao, D., Young, S. L., & Golden, C. D. (2015). A meta-analysis of pica and micronutrient status. *American Journal of Human Biology*, *27*(1), 84–93. DOI: 10.1002/ajhb.22598 PMID: 25156147

Micali, N., De Stavola, B., Ploubidis, G., Simonoff, E., Treasure, J., & Field, A. E. (2015). Adolescent eating disorder behaviours and cognitions: Gender-specific effects of child, maternal and family risk factors. *The British Journal of Psychiatry*, *207*(4), 320–327. DOI: 10.1192/bjp.bp.114.152371 PMID: 26206865

Nicholls-Clow, R., Simmonds-Buckley, M., & Waller, G. (2024). Avoidant/restrictive food intake disorder: Systematic review and meta-analysis demonstrating the impact of study quality on prevalence rates. *Clinical Psychology Review*, *114*, 102502. DOI: 10.1016/j.cpr.2024.102502 PMID: 39298990

Pike, K. M., So, M., Hilbert, A., Maekawa, H., Shimanouchi, T., Wilfley, D., Dohm, F., Fairburn, C. G., & Weissman, R. S. (2021). Risk factors for anorexia nervosa and bulimia nervosa in Japan and compared to a U.S. sample. *International Journal of Eating Disorders*, *54*(2), 155–167. DOI: 10.1002/eat.23442 PMID: 33355934

Placek, C. D. (2017). Ethnomedical and sociocultural factors of pica substances in rural South India. *Ecology of Food and Nutrition*, *56*(3), 238–255. DOI: 10.1080/03670244.2017.1311255 PMID: 28418723

Qian, J., Wu, Y., Liu, F., Zhu, Y., Jin, H., Zhang, H., Wan, Y., Li, C., & Yu, D. (2022). An update on the prevalence of eating disorders in the general population: A systematic review and meta-analysis. *Eating and Weight Disorders*, *27*(2), 415–428. DOI: 10.1007/s40519-021-01162-z PMID: 33834377

Quiles Marcos, Y., Quiles Sebastián, M. J., Pamies Aubalat, L., Botella Ausina, J., & Treasure, J. (2013). Peer and family influence in eating disorders: A meta-analysis. *European Psychiatry : the Journal of the Association of European Psychiatrists*, *28*(4), 199–206. DOI: 10.1016/j.eurpsy.2012.03.005 PMID: 22944338

Rodgers, R. F., Berry, R., & Franko, D. L. (2018). Eating disorders in ethnic minorities: An update. *Current Psychiatry Reports*, *20*(10), 90. DOI: 10.1007/s11920-018-0938-3 PMID: 30155577

Ruchkin, V., Isaksson, J., Schwab-Stone, M., & Stickley, A. (2021). Prevalence and early risk factors for bulimia nervosa symptoms in inner-city youth: Gender and ethnicity perspectives. *Journal of Eating Disorders*, *9*(1), 136. DOI: 10.1186/s40337-021-00479-5 PMID: 34674763

Sader, M., Weston, A., Buchan, K., Kerr-Gaffney, J., Gillespie-Smith, K., Sharpe, H., & Duffy, F. (2025). The co-occurrence of autism and avoidant/restrictive food intake disorder (ARFID): A prevalence-based meta-analysis. *International Journal of Eating Disorders*, *58*(3), 473–488. Advance online publication. DOI: 10.1002/eat.24369 PMID: 39760303

Schaefer, L. M., Burke, N. L., & Thompson, J. K. (2019). Thin-ideal internalization: How much is too much? *Eating and Weight Disorders*, *24*(5), 933–937. DOI: 10.1007/s40519-018-0498-x PMID: 29549566

Steiger, H., & Booij, L. (2020). Eating disorders, heredity and environmental activation: Getting epigenetic concepts into practice. *Journal of Clinical Medicine*, *9*(5), 1332. DOI: 10.3390/jcm9051332 PMID: 32375223

Steinhausen, H. C., Jakobsen, H., Helenius, D., Munk-Jørgensen, P., & Strober, M. (2015). A nation-wide study of the family aggregation and risk factors in anorexia nervosa over three generations. *International Journal of Eating Disorders*, *48*(1), 1–8. DOI: 10.1002/eat.22293 PMID: 24777686

Stice, E., Gau, J. M., Rohde, P., & Shaw, H. (2017). Risk factors that predict future onset of each *DSM–5* eating disorder: Predictive specificity in high-risk adolescent females. *Journal of Abnormal Psychology*, *126*(1), 38–51. DOI: 10.1037/abn0000219 PMID: 27709979

Van Dyne, A., Washington, N., Villodas, M., & Cronan, T. (2023). Racial/ethnic differences in anorexia and bulimia diagnoses among U.S. college students. *Eating Behaviors*, *50*, 101779. DOI: 10.1016/j.eatbeh.2023.101779 PMID: 37418803

Yamamiya, Y., & Stice, E. (2024). Risk factors that predict future onset of anorexia nervosa, bulimia nervosa, binge eating disorder, and purging disorder in adolescent girls. *Behavior Therapy, 55*(4), 712–723. DOI: 10.1016/j.beth.2023.10.002 PMID: 38937045

Zanella, E., & Lee, E. (2022). Integrative review on psychological and social risk and prevention factors of eating disorders including anorexia nervosa and bulimia nervosa: Seven major theories. *Heliyon, 8*(11), e11422. DOI: 10.1016/j.heliyon.2022.e11422 PMID: 36406673

Zimmerman, J., & Fisher, M. (2017). Avoidant/restrictive food intake disorder (ARFID). *Current Problems in Pediatric and Adolescent Health Care, 47*(4), 95–103. DOI: 10.1016/j.cppeds.2017.02.005 PMID: 28532967

KEY TERMS AND DEFINITIONS

Body Dissatisfaction: Negative thoughts and feelings someone has about their body shape or size, which can lead to disordered behaviors.

Emotion Dysregulation: Difficulties coping with strong emotions like stress, sadness, or anger.

Familial Risk Factors: Traits or problems within the family environment, such as high expectations or poor communication patterns, which increase the risk of a disorder, including an eating disorder.

Internalization of the Thin Ideal: A phenomenon that occurs when a person believes that being thin is desirable and necessary to be accepted and valued, in line with cultural messages.

Media Influence: Refers to the fact that social media, advertisements, and mainstream entertainment tend to promote unrealistic body standards.

Perfectionism: The tendency to set unrealistically high expectations for oneself and feel intense negative emotions when these standards are not met.

Sociocultural Pressures: Forces from larger society, such as cultural norms or peer expectations, that affect how people believe they should look or behave.

Chapter 3
History of Eating Disorder Treatment

ABSTRACT

This chapter traces the history of eating disorder treatment, exploring its evolution from early descriptions in historical texts to modern integrated, evidence-based approaches. Beginning with self-starvation in medieval times, the chapter covers the recognition and medicalization of eating disorders during the Renaissance and early 20th century. It examines the development of psychoanalytic, behavioral, and cognitive therapies, highlighting the shift toward evidence-based options like CBT and DBT. Addressing contemporary challenges, the chapter also discusses personalized medicine, telehealth, and disparities in access to care.

INTRODUCTION

Eating disorders have long posed significant challenges to public health, due to their complex etiologies and severe health implications. However, we have not always understood eating disorders the way that we do today. Understanding the historical progression of eating disorder treatment provides valuable insights into contemporary evidence-based practices and highlights the substantial progress made in addressing these disorders. This chapter highlights how the understanding and treatment of eating disorders has evolved over time, paving the way for the treatment strategies clinicians use today.

DOI 10.4018/979-8-3373-0664-3.ch003

EARLY HISTORICAL PERSPECTIVES ON EATING DISORDERS

Eating disorders have not always been classified exactly as they are in today's diagnostic manuals, but historical records reveal that behaviors resembling modern-day eating disorders have been recognized for centuries. For example, during the Middle ages, the term "anorexia mirabilis" was given to describe a spiritual practice, more commonly seen in women, that involved self-starvation. During this time, Catherina from Siena was known to have died prematurely from self-induced starvation. In some instances, self-starvation during this period was attributed to demonic possession, but some women were seen as being holy because of their severe food restriction (Dell'Osso et al., 2016).

The narrative related to self-starvation began to change during the Renaissance, when the explanation for this behavior moved beyond spirituality and became more appearance-related. During this time, society also adopted more of a medical explanation for behaviors related to anorexia. By the end of the 18th century, Morton had published the book "Phthisiologia or a Treatise of Consumptions," which referenced a condition called "nervous atrophy," which involved restriction of food intake. The cause of nervous atrophy was believed to be psychological (Dell'Osso et al., 2016).

As society has evolved, there has also been a shift in the ideal, feminine body type. While rounder female bodies were once valued, by the middle of the 18th century, a slender female figure became the cultural ideal, representing wealth and prosperity. The preference for thinness continued into the 19th century, when art featured tall, thin female figures, known for strict diets and strenuous exercise regimens. The preference for a slender female physique continues in modern times, with the diet industry equating thinness with health, and Western ideals pressuring women to maintain a slender body (Dell'Osso et al., 2016).

FORMAL RECOGNITION OF EATING DISORDERS

By the end of the 1800s, anorexia nervosa was recognized as a psychological condition, and eventually, it was the first eating disorder included in the original *Diagnostic and Statistical Manual of Mental Disorders (DSM).* Anorexia was initially considered a neurotic illness, but by the second publication of the *DSM,* it was classified as a feeding disturbance, alongside pica and rumination disorder. The third edition of the *DSM* classified eating disorders as disorders of childhood and adolescence, which was problematic, as cases emerging later i life were often missed. Eating disorders were included as an independent chapter in a text-revised 4th edition of the *DSM* (Dell'Osso et al., 2016).

EARLY 20th CENTURY APPROACHES TO EATING DISORDER TREATMENT

Around the same time that anorexia nervosa earned formal recognition as a psychological disorder, Sigmund Freud was fathering the psychoanalytic approach to therapy, which focused on how subconscious thoughts control the conscious mind and impede functioning. This approach would have been applicable to eating disorder treatment, because eating behaviors may be a cover for deeper, unconscious psychological issues (Tian, 2023). The application of psychoanalytic therapy to eating disorders began in the late 19th and early 20th centuries, building upon earlier medical observations. While initial medical descriptions of conditions like anorexia nervosa were provided by physicians such as Louis-Victor Marcé, Sir William Gull, and Ernest-Charles Lasègue, the psychoanalytic perspective emerged subsequently, focusing on the psychological underpinnings of these disorders (Farrell, 1995).

Sigmund Freud had made earlier connections between eating behaviors and psychological states. In his 1905 work, "Three Essays on the Theory of Sexuality," Freud discussed the oral phase of psychosexual development, linking nourishment and sexuality. He suggested that disturbances during this phase could manifest in behaviors related to eating and sexuality. In the early 20th century, other psychoanalysts expanded upon Freud's ideas. Pierre Janet, in 1903, documented bulimic behaviors in his patients, noting the psychological aspects of these eating patterns. Similarly, physicians like William Osler and L. Vernon Riddle, in the early 1900s, linked symptoms of food cravings and vomiting to hysteria, further exploring the psychological dimensions of eating disorders. These early psychoanalytic contributions laid the groundwork for understanding eating disorders as complex conditions influenced by both physiological and psychological factors. This perspective shaped the way eating disorders were treated in the earlier days, and its evolution has significantly shaped modern therapeutic approaches to treating eating disorders (Farrell, 1995).

SHIFTS DURING THE MID-20th CENTURY

Shortly after psychoanalytic approaches became popular, behavioral therapy took center stage. This treatment modality became popular in the 1950s, after animal research revealed that using rewards and punishments could shape behavior. Behavioral interventions were only moderately effective for addressing eating disorder symptoms, so further exploration continued. Researchers became interested in the use of psychiatric medications for treating eating disorder symptoms, and they found that antidepressant and antipsychotic medications were beneficial for short-term mood stabilization. Unfortunately, these medications showed little benefit for normalizing weight and eating behaviors (Binh & Huong, 2024), so there was more work to be done.

Behavioral and pharmaceutical methods may not have been entirely effective for treating eating disorder symptoms, but the cognitive revolution in the late 1950s and early 1960s offered a different perspective. The revolution began when Albert Ellis, a psychotherapist, recognized that distorted thinking patterns were at the center of many client problems. Ellis developed Rational-Emotive Therapy, which eventually became Rational-Emotive Behavior Therapy (REBT) as a departure from psychoanalysis, which he found to be too slow to produce progress. Ellis focused on helping clients replace irrational thinking patterns with more rational thought processes that promoted mental wellness. Aaron Beck built upon Ellis' ideas, developing cognitive therapy, which focused on correcting automatic negative thoughts (Dowd, 2004). During the cognitive revolution, cognitive behavioral therapy (CBT) emerged as a method for correcting irrational thinking patterns related to eating disorders. For instance, CBT sought to correct distorted cognitions, such as poor body image, rigidity, and the insistence on perfection, which often occur with eating disorders (Binh & Huong, 2024).

THE RISE OF EVIDENCE-BASED TREATMENT IN EATING DISORDERS (LATE 20th-21st CENUTRY)

Throughout the 1980s, eating disorder treatment remained somewhat disjointed. Experts understood that the best treatment approach was integrated and involved psychological, medical, family-based, and nutritional treatments, but approaches at the time failed to be truly integrated. Nonetheless, early approaches, including behavioral interventions, use of medication, and CBT, showed just how complex eating disorders were, which set the stage for the evidence-based treatment programs used today. At the end of the 20th century and continuing into the early 21st century, new eating disorder treatment programs were explored. For instance, hospitals have implemented treatment programs that not only offer weight restoration and medical supervision but also involve family in the treatment process. Interventions specific to eating disorders, such as enhanced cognitive behavioral therapy (CBT-E), have also emerged. Dialectical behavior therapy (DBT), with its focus on emotion regulation, has also shown promise for eating disorder treatment (Binh & Huong, 2024). The ultimate goal of exploring new treatment modalities via research is to promote evidence-based practice (EBP). Principles of EBP call upon practitioners to select interventions that are based on positive research outcomes, while also considering their own clinical expertise and client preferences (National Association of Social Workers, n.d.).

CONTEMPORARY TREATMENT APPROACHES AND FUTURE DIRECTIONS

Exploration of evidence-based eating disorder approaches continues today. Contemporary treatment approaches integrate neurobiological research, recognizing the role of brain function and genetics in eating disorders. Personalized medicine tailors interventions to individual genetic and psychological profiles, which improves treatment effectiveness for each patient (Kaye, 2009). In addition, emerging research into the gut-brain axis and nutritional psychiatry explores how diet influences mental health, potentially informing novel treatment strategies for eating disorders (Cryan & Dinan, 2012).

Beyond exploration into novel strategies for intervention, practitioners have become interested in new treatment delivery methods. In recent years, digital and telehealth interventions have expanded access to care, offering remote therapy options that are especially valuable in underserved areas. During the COVID-19 pandemic, research revealed that telehealth interventions could feasibly be implemented to treat adolescent eating disorders. There is continued interest in hybrid treatment methods, which are likely to continue in the aftermath of the pandemic, but ongoing research is necessary to determine best practices (Gorrell et al., 2022).

Despite recent advancements in eating disorder treatment, challenges persist in ensuring equitable access to care and addressing treatment disparities across different populations. These disparities, and the evidence base of current treatment approaches, are discussed more fully in future chapters.

REFERENCES

Binh, T. T. N., & Huong, X. V. (2024). Eating disorders: A historical perspective and analysis of current treatment approaches. *International Journal of Innovative Research in Multidisciplinary Education, 3*(4), 513–519. DOI: 10.58806/ijirme.2024.v3i4n07

Cryan, J. F., & Dinan, T. G. (2012). Mind-altering microorganisms: The impact of the gut microbiota on brain and behaviour. *Nature Reviews. Neuroscience, 13*(10), 701–712. DOI: 10.1038/nrn3346 PMID: 22968153

Dell'Osso, L., Abelli, M., Carpita, B., Pini, S., Castellini, G., Carmassi, C., & Ricca, V. (2016).

Dowd, E. T. (2004). Cognition and the cognitive revolution in psychotherapy: Promises and advances. *Journal of Clinical Psychology, 60*(4), 415–428. DOI: 10.1002/jclp.10253 PMID: 15022271

Farrell, E. (1995). Psychoanalytic understanding. In Young, R. M. (Ed.), *Lost for words: The psychoanalysis of anorexia and bulimia*. Psychoanalysis and Psychotherapy., Retrieved from https://www.psychoanalysis-and-therapy.com/human_nature/farrell/chap2.html

Gorrell, S., Reilly, E. E., Brosof, L., & Le Grange, D. (2022). Use of telehealth in the management of adolescent eating disorders: Patient perspectives and future directions suggested from the COVID-19 pandemic. *Adolescent Health, Medicine and Therapeutics, 13*, 45–53. DOI: 10.2147/AHMT.S334977 PMID: 35401019

Kaye, W. H., Fudge, J. L., & Paulus, M. (2009). New insights into symptoms and neurocircuit function of anorexia nervosa. *Nature Reviews. Neuroscience, 10*(8), 573–584. DOI: 10.1038/nrn2682 PMID: 19603056

National Association of Social Workers. (n.d.). *Evidence-based practice*. NASW. https://www.socialworkers.org/News/Research-Data/Social-Work-Policy-Research/Evidence-Based-Practice

Pini, S., Abelli, M., Carpita, B., Dell'Osso, L., Castellini, G., Carmassi, C., & Ricca, V. (2016, July). Historical evolution of the concept of anorexia nervosa and relationships with orthorexia nervosa, autism, and obsessive–compulsive spectrum. *Neuropsychiatric Disease and Treatment*, *12*, 1651–1660. DOI: 10.2147/NDT.S108912 PMID: 27462158

Tian, Z. (2023). Understanding and treating eating disorders in a psychoanalytic approach. *Proceedings of the 4th International Conference on Educational Innovation and Philosophical Inquiries*. https://doi.org/ DOI: 10.54254/2753-7048/18/20231276

KEY TERMS AND DEFINITIONS

Anorexia Mirabilis: A term from the Middle Ages, used to describe a spiritual practice, mostly employed by women, that involved self-starvation.

Behavioral Therapy: An approach focused on using rewards and punishments to influence behavior.

Cognitive Therapy: Aaron Beck's therapeutic model, which emphasizes correcting automatic negative thoughts.

Diagnostic and Statistical Manual of Mental Disorders (DSM): The original diagnostic manual that included criteria for diagnosing various mental disorders, including anorexia nervosa.

Evidence-Based Practice: Refers to the use of research evidence, client preferences, and clinical expertise when choosing interventions for clients.

Nervous Atrophy: A Renaissance-era term used to describe psychologically-based food restriction.

Psychoanalytic Approach: A therapeutic modality developed by Sigmund Freud, which emphasized the role of subconscious thoughts in creating psychological dysfunction.

Rational Emotive Behavior Therapy: An approach developed by Albert Ellis, which focused on altering irrational thinking patterns.

Section 2
Specific Eating Disorder Treatment Modalities

Chapter 4 Systematic Review of Eating Disorder Treatment

ABSTRACT

This chapter provides a review of evidence-based treatments for eating disorders as classified in the DSM-5-TR. Each disorder is examined individually, beginning with anorexia nervosa, where treatment varies by age—family-based approaches are preferred for adolescents, while adults benefit from a combination of psychotherapies and nutritional support. For bulimia nervosa, cognitive behavioral therapy (CBT) is the most widely supported treatment for adults, with family-based approaches also showing effectiveness in adolescents. Binge-eating disorder is primarily treated with CBT, though interpersonal therapy, pharmacological interventions, and behavioral weight loss programs offer additional options. Treatment of avoidant/restrictive food intake disorder (ARFID) requires family interventions. Rumination disorder is typically managed through behavioral techniques like diaphragmatic breathing and biofeedback. Pica is treated primarily through behavioral interventions, with pharmacological and nutritional supplements used in select cases, particularly where comorbidities exist.

DOI: 10.4018/979-8-3373-0664-3.ch004

INTRODUCTION

As discussed in the previous chapter, the understanding of eating disorders and their treatment has evolved over time. As our understanding of evidence-based practices has grown, a rather large base of research knowledge has been established. This chapter will provide a brief systematic review of evidence-based eating disorder treatments, with each eating disorder in the DSM-5-TR discussed separately. A keyword searched was performed to identify research related to evidence-based treatments for each respective disorder, and relevant articles published within the last 10 years were included in the systematic review; some articles were themselves systematic reviews. Once material became redundant, no additional articles were reviewed. The purpose of this chapter is to set the stage for a more detailed discussion of specific treatment modalities in future chapters, and to provide a general overview of how professionals treat each eating disorder.

EVIDENCE-BASED PRACTICES FOR ANOREXIA NERVOSA

The best treatment for anorexia nervosa may depend upon the patient's age. Family-based interventions have been identified as effective for adolescents living with anorexia. However, for adults, there is not one specific treatment modality that has emerged as most effective. Instead, some combination of refeeding approaches and psychotherapy seems to be beneficial (Zipfel et al., 2015).

Research into more specific treatment approaches has found that there is strong support for family-based treatment, and even more specifically, Maudsley Family Therapy, for adolescent patients with anorexia nervosa. There is also moderate evidence supporting family system therapy and cognitive behavioral approaches, especially enhanced cognitive behavioral treatment (CBT). Furthermore, outpatient family therapy is beneficial for preventing relapse after hospitalization in adolescents (Brockmeyer et al., 2018). The evidence base is not as strong for adults, according to a review of the research. There is moderate evidence supporting enhanced

CBT for adults, as well as moderate evidence for some psychodynamic approaches and for the Maudsley model of anorexia nervosa treatment for adults (MANTRA). Some psychodynamic approaches for adults show only weak evidence, and broad cognitive behavioral approaches are also weak. Interpersonal and behavioral therapies for adult anorexia have a weak evidence base, and behavioral therapy may even be harmful. Finally, specialist supportive clinical management shows moderate beneficial effects for adult anorexia (Zipfel et al., 2015).

A recent research review found that both enhanced CBT and psychodynamic therapy have benefits for adults with anorexia. Weight gain occurs more rapidly for enhanced CBT compared to psychodynamic therapy, but psychodynamic methods appear to be more cost-effective. Furthermore, psychodynamic therapy, enhanced CBT and treatment as usual are all equally effective for increasing BMI, despite the fact that weight gain occurs more quickly with enhanced CBT. Additional research has found that MANTRA, specialist supportive clinical management, and enhanced CBT are equally effective for treating adult anorexia, with none of these methods emerging as superior to the others. Finally, a small body of research shows that exposure therapy may be beneficial for anorexia in adults. Exposure therapies using food exposure can increase calorie intake and alleviate anxiety at mealtimes, which can be beneficial for recovery (Brockmeyer et al., 2018).

Additional research has revealed that enhanced CBT is effective for treating severe, enduring cases of anorexia in inpatient settings. This treatment modality is beneficial for increasing BMI and improving general and eating disorder pathology. Some evidence suggests that enhanced CBT is superior to specialist supportive clinical management, because CBT promotes better social adjustment and reduces eating disorder symptoms more significantly (Marcolini et al., 2024). However, this is in conflict with earlier research showing that enhanced CBT was not superior to specialist supportive clinical management (Brockmeyer et al., 2018). Nonetheless, both treatment options have demonstrated effectiveness for treating anorexia nervosa.

Beyond the psychotherapies discussed above, alternative treatment modalities, including brain stimulation and medication, have received interest in recent years. The antipsychotic olanzapine may be beneficial for promoting weight gain, but it doesn't tend to improve psychological symptoms (Brockmeyer, 2018; Marcolini et al., 2024). The antipsychotic medication haloperidol has also been identified as beneficial for promoting weight gain and reducing body image disturbances. Furthermore, the synthetic cannabinoid dronabinal may promote weight gain, but some research has found that it does not have significant benefits for patients with anorexia (Marcolini et al., 2024). Some individuals living with anorexia nervosa may benefit from the use of medications to supplement gains made through psychotherapy.

In addition, experts have taken interest in cognitive remediation therapy. This modality aims to enhance cognitive functioning using exercises that address areas like cognitive flexibility, to overcome issues like extreme attention to detail, which are seen in individuals with anorexia nervosa. Preliminary research shows that cognitive remediation therapy can improve neural correlates of poor cognitive flexibility in patients with anorexia nervosa. On the other hand, some research has not found cognitive remediation therapy to be beneficial, and additional studies are needed. Similarly, some forms of brain stimulation have shown promise for treating anorexia nervosa, but additional research, particularly in the form of randomized controlled trials, is warranted (Brockmeyer et al., 2018). A recent narrative review did conclude that transcranial direct current stimulation (tDCS), a non-invasive brain stimulation technique, can improve clinical symptoms of anorexia, but research is still limited (Chmiel et al., 2023).

Finally, nutritional interventions form a cornerstone of anorexia nervosa treatment, especially for severely underweight or malnourished patients. The goal of nutritional interventions is to promote weight gain and correct malnutrition, while also normalizing eating patterns. Ultimately, nutritional interventions are considered successful when they result in a healthy weight for the patient. For women, this can be defined as a return to menstruation and ovulation; for men, a healthy weight can be operationalized as a normalization of sexual desire and hormone levels. In children and adolescents, nutritional interventions are deemed successful when normal growth and sexual development resume (Cuerda et al., 2019).

Unfortunately, there is limited data from randomized controlled trials of nutritional interventions in anorexia nervosa, but there is evidence based on clinical experience. Nutritional interventions should provide refeeding, which aims to increase calorie intake to promote weight gain. Both the American Psychological Association and the American Dietetic Association recommend beginning the refeeding process with 30-40 kcal/kilogram of body weight per day. Calorie intake should increase over time to promote continued weight gain, and patients should also be provided with electrolyte, vitamin, and mineral supplementation. There is some evidence that patients with lower BMIs benefit from a refeeding process that begins slowly, whereas those with a higher body weight benefit from a faster process. Refeeding can occur via oral diet, and nutritional supplements can be added, as needed, if oral diet alone is not sufficient. Patients who refuse to eat may require tube feeding (Cuerda et al, 2019).

In summary, this brief systematic review underscores that effective treatment modalities for anorexia nervosa vary based on patient age and specific needs. For adolescents, family-based interventions, particularly Maudsley Family Therapy, demonstrate strong efficacy in promoting weight restoration and preventing relapse (Brockmeyer et al., 2018). In adults, while no single psychotherapy emerges as universally superior, approaches such as enhanced cognitive behavioral therapy (CBT-E), the Maudsley Model of Anorexia Nervosa Treatment for Adults (MANTRA), and specialist supportive clinical management have shown moderate effectiveness (Zipfel et al., 2015). Emerging treatments, including cognitive remediation therapy and non-invasive brain stimulation techniques like transcranial direct current stimulation (tDCS), offer promising avenues but require further research to establish their efficacy (Brockmeyer et al., 2018; Chmiel et al., 2023). Pharmacological interventions, such as the use of olanzapine and haloperidol, may support weight gain but often lack significant impact on psychological symptoms (Marcolini et al., 2024). Nutritional interventions are also often necessary to restore weight and correct nutritional deficiencies (Cuerda et al., 2019). These findings highlight the importance of individualized, multidisciplinary treatment strategies, integrating both established and novel therapies, to address the complex and multifaceted nature of anorexia nervosa.

EVIDENCE-BASED PRACTICES FOR BULIMIA NERVOSA

Some evidence-based treatments for bulimia nervosa align with treatments for anorexia nervosa, but there are also some differences in preferred treatments for the two disorders. According to a meta-analysis of the effectiveness of different bulimia treatments, CBT specific to eating disorders is the most effective for achieving remission of bulimia symptoms in adults (Hagan & Walsh, 2021; Slade et al., 2018). Guided CBT self-help programs are also effective for treating bulimia nervosa. While CBT, including self-help versions, have been found to be effective for treatment of bulimia in adults, there is also evidence that interpersonal therapy, dialectical behavior therapy, and cognitive-affective therapy are beneficial. Group behavioral therapy is also beneficial, and it has been found to be superior to interpersonal therapy and individual behavioral therapy, but the evidence is based on small sample sizes, so further research is warranted (Slade at al., 2019).

For adolescents with bulimia nervosa, both family-based interventions and CBT are beneficial, according to research (Hagan & Walsh, 2021; Hail & Le Grange, 2018). However, there is an overall lack of research on evidence-based treatments for youth living with bulimia. The current evidence suggests that involving the family in treatment is beneficial, but it is essential for researchers to continue to add to the evidence base for bulimia treatments (Hail & Le Grange, 2018).

Medication may beneficial for treating bulimia, but the best practice is to utilize medication alongside psychotherapy. The selective serotonin reuptake inhibitor (SSRI) fluoxetine is the first pharmacological treatment of choice for bulimia in adults. There isn't as much evidence for pharmacological treatments for bulimia in adolescents, but fluoxetine may also be beneficial for this population (Hagan & Walsh, 2021).

Based on brief systematic review, there are some evidence-based treatments for bulimia nervosa—primarily CBT for adults and family-based treatments for adolescents—but there is an overall paucity of research related to treatments for this eating disorder (Hagan & Walsh, 2021; Slade et al., 2018). More rigorous, controlled studies are warranted to clarify the best practices for treating bulimia nervosa. Continued investigation into both psychotherapeutic and pharmacological interventions is essential, especially for younger populations.

EVIDENCE-BASED PRACTICES FOR BINGE-EATING DISORDER

Meta-analytic research with binge eating disorder has revealed that psychotherapy, and specifically CBT, is beneficial for reducing binge-eating behavior. Self-help programs based on principles from CBT are also effective, but psychotherapy is superior to self-help for promoting long-term abstinence from binge-eating. CBT also emerges as superior to other counseling modalities, including interpersonal therapy, psychodynamic therapy, and humanistic therapy, for reducing binge-eating (Hilbert et al., 2019). CBT is so beneficial for treating binge-eating disorder that it is typically seen as the first line of treatment for this eating disorder; numerous systematic reviews and meta analyses have demonstrated the effectiveness of CBT in populations with binge-eating disorder (da Luz et al., 2020; Grilo, 2017).

CBT is often considered the gold standard for psychotherapy in patients with binge-eating disorder; however, it is not the only effective modality utilized with this population. For example, research with interpersonal psychotherapy has revealed that this modality produces 50-60% remission rates, as defined by abstinence from binge-eating. Some research has even found that interpersonal psychotherapy is more effective than CBT for promoting abstinence from binge-eating (Linardon, 2018). Preliminary evidence also suggests that dialectical behavior therapy, with its focus on emotion regulation and distress tolerance, may be beneficial for reducing binge-eating (Grilo, 2017).

Beyond psychotherapies, binge-eating disorder may also be responsive to pharmacological interventions. Second generation antidepressants, including fluvoxamine, and the central nervous stimulant lisdexamfetamine are commonly used in treatment of binge-eating disorder. Both types of medications have benefits, but they may be more effective when used in combination with CBT. Medications may have side effects that lead to discontinuation (Hilbert et al., 2019). Among the pharmacological options for treatment of BPD, lisdexamfetamine, known by the brand name Vyvanse, is the only option with FDA approval specifically for the treatment of binge-eating disorder. The medication is well-tolerated in individuals with moderate to severe binge eating disorder. Clinical trials have also demonstrated that the medication is effective for reducing binge eating days as well as preventing relapse to binge-eating (Heo & Duggan, 2017).

While lisdexamfetamine is the only FDA-approved medication for binge-eating disorder as of the writing of this textbook, pilot studies are currently underway to assess the effectiveness of the glucagon-like peptide-1 (GLP1) analog semaglutide for treating binge-eating disorder. One study found that semaglutide may be more effective than topiramate, which is prescribed off-label for binge-eating disorder, in addition to being superior to lisdexamfetamine. However, additional research with semaglutide is needed to confirm its benefits for treating binge-eating disorder (Richards et al., 2023).

Some binge eating disorder treatment programs use behavioral weight loss interventions. For instance, the Health Approach to Weight Management and Food in Eating Disorders (HAPIFED) program promotes healthy weight loss in individuals with binge-eating disorder by helping individuals to create home environments that support weight loss. It also teaches skills like creating new routines and engaging in physical activity. The program also includes educational components, such as learning about the health risks associated with high body weight, the symptoms of eating disorders, and the way that mood states can lead to binge eating. In a clinical trial, HAPIFED was found to be equally effective when compared to enhanced cognitive behavioral therapy (CBT) on the whole. However, it was more effective than CBT for promoting remission from binge eating (Palavras et al., 2021).

While the clinical trial with HAPIFED showed that this behavioral weight loss intervention was more effective than CBT for promoting remission from binge eating, other research shows that behavioral weight less treatment tends to be less effective than psychotherapy modalities, including CBT. Nonetheless, behavioral weight loss treatment, which aims to both increase physical activity and normalize eating patterns, is effective for promoting moderate weight loss while also reducing binging behavior

(Grilo, 2017). The HAPIFED program is not the only behavioral weight loss intervention available. There are a wide variety of interventions under this umbrella, but all aim to create a balanced lifestyle, in which patients maintain structured eating patterns involving moderate calorie reduction and improved nutritional content, as well as sustainable increases in physical activity. One randomized controlled trial found that behavioral weight loss interventions yielded remission rates around 50%, which is similar to the remission rate seen with CBT and interpersonal psychotherapy. The added benefit of behavioral weight loss interventions is that they result in sustained weight loss, which can be beneficial given the link between binge-eating disorder and weight-related metabolic comorbidities (Grilo & Juarascio, 2023).

In summary, while several treatment options exist for binge-eating disorder, CBT consistently emerges as the most effective and widely supported intervention, serving as the first-line treatment due to its robust empirical backing (Hilbert et al., 2019; Grilo, 2017). Nonetheless, interpersonal psychotherapy and dialectical behavior therapy also demonstrate meaningful clinical outcomes, with IPT occasionally outperforming CBT in promoting abstinence (Linardon, 2018). Pharmacological treatments, particularly lisdexamfetamine, offer additional support, especially when integrated with psychotherapy, although side effects and long-term adherence should be considered (Heo & Duggan, 2017). Moreover, behavioral weight loss interventions like the HAPIFED program provide an alternative approach that not only reduces binge-eating episodes but also addresses metabolic health concerns, showing comparable remission rates to psychotherapeutic interventions (Palavras et al., 2021; Grilo & Juarascio, 2023). As the field advances, promising treatments like semaglutide may expand future options, but continued research is needed to validate their effectiveness and safety (Richards et al., 2023).

EVIDENCE-BASED PRACTICES FOR AVOIDANT-RESTRICTIVE FOOD INTAKE DISORDER (ARFID)

Treatment approaches for ARFID must address malnutrition and poor weight gain, in addition to treating the underlying psychological factors contributing to food aversion. In cases where an individual's health is at risk from poor nutritional status, this must be addressed first, before treating underlying psychological factors. For children and young adults, parenting and family-based interventions are often the treatment of choice. Such interventions can provide parents with strategies for reducing conflict, managing mealtimes, and introducing new foods to children (Archibald & Bryant-Waugh, 2023). Researchers have recently conducted pilot studies with a specific parenting program called Supportive Parenting for Anxious Childhood Emotions adapted for avoidant/restrictive food intake disorder (SPACE-ARFID), and results showed that both parents and children found the program satisfactory. Additionally, ARFID severity and impairment from the disorder declined significantly after program participation (Shimshoni et al., 2020).

In addition to parenting and family-based programs, individuals with ARFID often benefit from dietetic, medical, and pharmacological interventions. Dietetic interventions may involve presenting preferred foods while gradually introducing feared foods. This is particularly beneficial for those with sensory aversion to foods. Those who lack interest in eating benefit from interventions aimed at creating structured mealtime routines and providing rewards for eating. When ARFID involves lack of interest in eating, it is also helpful to include the person in food shopping and meal preparation. In addition to the aforementioned interventions, patients with ARFID may require supplements to address deficiencies. Medical and pharmacological treatments may also include medications to alleviate constipation or stimulate the appetite. Furthermore, food anxiety may improve with medications including buspirone, lorazepam, or fluoxetine. That being said, medication is typically not the first line of treatment, and additional research is needed to confirm best practices for pharmacological management of ARFID (Archibald & Bryant-Waugh, 2023).

Among the psychotherapy options for ARFID, there is not one modality that emerges as most effective. Cognitive-behavioral (CBT), family-based, and behavioral treatments appear to be most promising. Some CBT interventions have been adapted specifically for treatment of ARFID (Archibald & Bryant-Waugh, 2023; Willmott et al., 2024). Unfortunately, much of the evidence base for psychological treatments for ARFID is based on small, low-quality studies, so additional research is necessary (Willmott et al., 2024).

Based on current research evidence, effective treatment for avoidant/restrictive food intake disorder (ARFID) requires addressing both nutritional deficiencies and the psychological factors underlying food avoidance. In medically severe cases, nutritional stabilization must come first. Family-based approaches, such as SPACE-ARFID, have shown promise in reducing symptom severity and improving parental involvement (Shimshoni et al., 2020; Archibald & Bryant-Waugh, 2023). Dietetic strategies like gradual food exposure and structured mealtimes are helpful, especially for those with sensory sensitivities or low appetite. While medications may support treatment, they are not first-line interventions and require further study. Among psychotherapies, CBT, behavioral, and family-based treatments are most promising, though the current evidence base is limited and highlights the need for more high-quality research (Willmott et al., 2024).

EVIDENCE-BASED PRACTICES FOR RUMINATION DISORDER

The body of research related to evidence-based treatments for rumination disorder is sparse. In much of the literature, rumination disorder is treated as a gastrointestinal condition, called rumination syndrome. Current guidelines state that treatment must begin with a nutritional assessment to evaluate if a patient is at risk of malnutrition and in need of nutritional support. Beyond this, rumination disorder is primarily treated with behavioral interventions. Diaphragmatic breathing is useful for reducing regurgitation, and biofeedback can teach patients to relax the muscles in their abdominal wall after eating. Behavioral interventions may be supplemented with cognitive-behavioral therapy (CBT). There is limited research on pharmacological treatment of rumination disorder, but baclofen may be effective (Sasegbon et al., 2022).

EVIDENCE-BASED PRACTICES FOR PICA

Because pica involves the consumption of non-nutritive substances, it can be dangerous to one's health, and potentially fatal. Given this risk, behavioral interventions that stop the consumption of non-nutritive substances are essential. Research has found that behavioral interventions including contingent reinforcement for desired behavior can essentially eliminate pica. More restrictive behavioral interventions, such as punishment, should be utilized only when interventions like contingent reinforcement are not effective. Some research suggests that parents can be trained to perform behavioral interventions at home (Moline et al., 2021; Thomas et al., 2023). Discrimination training, in which the individual is taught to differentiate between food and non-food items can also be an effective behavioral intervention; however, many of the studies evaluating pica treatments are small, so there is limited research on best practices (Moline et al., 2021; Williams et al., 2022).

While behavioral interventions are the most common choice for treatment of pica, pharmacological treatment may also be used. Medication is not the first line of treatment but rather an option in cases in which there are comorbidities present. For instance, methylphenidate may be effective for treating pica in people with comorbid ADHD, according to case reports. Antipsychotic medications, bupropion, and mood stabilizers including lithium may also be efficacious for some patients. There is a lack of rigorous research with pharmacological interventions for pica, so medications should be used with caution (Williams et al., 2022).

Iron supplementation is another potential treatment for pica, especially in adults. There is evidence of a link between pica and iron deficiency anemia, so iron supplementation may eliminate symptoms in some patients. A recent research review found that treatment of iron deficiency led to resolution of pica symptoms (Ganesan & Vasauskas, 2023).

Finally, surgical interventions may be necessary in some cases, as consumption of non-food substances can cause perforations, blockages, or the formation of masses within the gastrointestinal tract. If surgery is necessary, it can prevent serious complications from pica, but it does not treat the underlying factors contributing to the disorder (Moline et al., 2021).

CONCLUSION

In conclusion, this chapter highlights the importance of individualized, evidence-based treatment approaches tailored to each eating disorder's unique features and patient demographics. For anorexia nervosa, treatments vary by age, with family-based therapy effective in adolescents and enhanced CBT, MANTRA, and specialist supportive clinical management offering moderate benefits for adults (Zipfel et al., 2015; Brockmeyer et al., 2018; Marcolini et al., 2024). Bulimia nervosa responds well to CBT, particularly in adults, with family-based therapy recommended for youth, though more research is needed in adolescent populations (Hagan & Walsh, 2021; Hail & Le Grange, 2018). Binge-eating disorder is best treated with CBT, though interpersonal psychotherapy, pharmacological options like lisdexamfetamine, and behavioral weight loss programs such as HAPIFED also show promise (Hilbert et al., 2019; Grilo & Juarascio, 2023; Palavras et al., 2021). ARFID treatment must address nutritional deficits first and combine dietary, psychological, and family-based strategies, though the evidence base remains limited (Archibald & Bryant-Waugh, 2023; Shimshoni et al., 2020; Willmott et al., 2024). For rumination disorder, behavioral interventions like diaphragmatic breathing remain the gold standard, with limited support for pharmacological treatment (Sasegbon et al., 2022). Lastly, pica treatment focuses on behavioral strategies, supplemented by pharmacological or nutritional interventions when indicated, especially in cases involving iron deficiency anemia or comorbidities (Moline et al., 2021; Williams et al., 2022; Ganesan & Vasauskas, 2023). Together, these findings emphasize the need for multidisciplinary, flexible treatment models grounded in both current research and clinical expertise. It is also evident that the field of eating disorder treatment would benefit from additional rigorous research to determine best practices.

REFERENCES

Archibald, T., & Bryant-Waugh, R. (2023). Current evidence for avoidant restrictive food intake disorder: Implications for clinical practice and future directions. *JCPP Advances*, *3*(2), e12160. DOI: 10.1002/jcv2.12160 PMID: 37753149

Brockmeyer, T., Friederich, H. C., & Schmidt, U. (2018). Advances in the treatment of anorexia nervosa: A review of established and emerging interventions. *Psychological Medicine*, *48*(8), 1228–1256. DOI: 10.1017/S0033291717002604 PMID: 28889819

Chmiel, J., Gladka, A., & Leszek, J. (2023). The effect of transcranial direct current stimulation (tDCS) on anorexia nervosa: A narrative review. *Nutrients*, *15*(20), 4455. DOI: 10.3390/nu15204455 PMID: 37892530

Cuerda, C., Vasiloglou, M. F., & Arhip, L. (2019). Nutritional management and outcomes in malnourished medical inpatients: Anorexia nervosa. *Journal of Clinical Medicine*, *8*(7), 1042. DOI: 10.3390/jcm8071042 PMID: 31319585

da Luz, F. Q., Hay, P., Wisniewski, L., Cordás, T., & Sainsbury, A. (2020). The treatment of binge eating disorder with cognitive behavior therapy and other therapies: An overview and clinical considerations. *Obesity Reviews*, *22*(5, S1), e13180. DOI: 10.1111/obr.13180 PMID: 33350574

Ganesan, P. R., & Vasauskas, A. A. (2023). The association between pica and iron-deficiency anemia: A scoping review. *Cureus*, *15*(4), e37904. DOI: 10.7759/cureus.37904 PMID: 37220446

Grilo, C. M. (2017). Psychological and behavioral treatments for binge-eating disorder. *The Journal of Clinical Psychiatry*, *78*(Suppl 1), 20–24. DOI: 10.4088/JCP.sh16003su1c.04 PMID: 28125175

Grilo, C. M., & Juarascio, A. (2023). Binge-eating disorder interventions: Review, current status, and implications. *Current Obesity Reports*, *12*(3), 406–416. DOI: 10.1007/s13679-023-00517-0 PMID: 37439970

Hagan, K. E., & Walsh, B. T. (2021). State of the art: The therapeutic approaches to bulimia nervosa. *Clinical Therapeutics*, *43*(1), 40–49. DOI: 10.1016/j.clinthera.2020.10.012 PMID: 33358256

Hail, L., & Le Grange, D. (2018). Bulimia nervosa in adolescents: Prevalence and treatment challenges. *Adolescent Health, Medicine and Therapeutics*, *9*, 11–16. DOI: 10.2147/AHMT.S135326 PMID: 29379324

Heo, Y.-A., & Duggan, S. T. (2017). Lisdexamfetamine: A review in binge eating disorder. *CNS Drugs*, *31*(11), 1015–1022. DOI: 10.1007/s40263-017-0477-1 PMID: 29134566

Hilbert, A., Petroff, D., Herpertz, S., Pietrowsky, R., Tuschen-Caffier, B., Vocks, S., & Schmidt, R. (2019). Meta-analysis of the efficacy of psychological and medical treatments for binge-eating disorder. *Journal of Consulting and Clinical Psychology*, *87*(1), 91–105. DOI: 10.1037/ccp0000358 PMID: 30570304

Linardon, J. (2018). Rates of abstinence following psychological or behavioral treatments for binge-eating disorder: Meta-analysis. *International Journal of Eating Disorders*, *51*(8), 785–797. DOI: 10.1002/eat.22897 PMID: 30058074

Marcolini, F., Ravaglia, A., Tempia Valenta, S., Bosco, G., Marconi, G., De Ronchi, D., & Atti, A. R. (2024). Severe enduring anorexia nervosa (SE-AN) treatment options and their effectiveness: A review of literature. *Journal of Eating Disorders*, *12*(48), 48. Advance online publication. DOI: 10.1186/s40337-024-01006-y PMID: 38654374

Moline, R., Hou, S., Chevrier, J., & Thomassin, K. (2021). A systematic review of the effectiveness of behavioural treatments for pica in youths. *Clinical Psychology & Psychotherapy*, *28*(1), 39–55. DOI: 10.1002/cpp.2491 PMID: 32628326

Palavras, M. A., Hay, P., Mannan, H., da Luz, F. Q., Sainsbury, A., Touyz, S., & Claudino, A. M. (2021). Integrated weight loss and cognitive behavioural therapy (CBT) for the treatment of recurrent binge eating and high body mass index: A randomized controlled trial. *Eating and Weight Disorders*, *26*(1), 249–262.

Richards, J., Bang, N., Ratliff, E. L., Paszkowiak, M. A., Khorgami, Z., Khalsa, S. S., & Simmons, W. K. (2023). Successful treatment of binge eating disorder with the GLP-1 agonist semaglutide: A retrospective cohort study. *Obesity Pillars*, *7*, 100080. DOI: 10.1016/j.obpill.2023.100080 PMID: 37990682

Sasegbon, A., Hasan, S. S., Disney, B. R., & Vasant, D. H. (2022). Rumination syndrome: Pathophysiology, diagnosis and practical management. *Frontline Gastroenterology*, *13*(5), 402–409. DOI: 10.1136/flgastro-2021-101856 PMID: 36046491

Shimshoni, Y., Silverman, W. K., & Lebowitz, E. R. (2020). SPACE-ARFID: A pilot trial of a novel parent-based treatment for avoidant/restrictive food intake disorder. *International Journal of Eating Disorders*, *53*(10), 1623–1635. DOI: 10.1002/eat.23341 PMID: 33464594

Slade, E., Keeney, E., Mavranezouli, I., Dias, S., Fou, L., Stockton, S., Saxon, L., Waller, G., Turner, H., Serpell, L., Fairburn, C. G., & Kendall, T. (2018). Treatments for bulimia nervosa: A network meta-analysis. *Psychological Medicine*, *48*(16), 2629–2636. DOI: 10.1017/S0033291718001071 PMID: 29729686

Thomas, B. R., Bowman, M. D., Sanchez, A., & Strohmeier, C. W. (2023). Parent treatment of complex pica in a teen with autism. *Behavioral Interventions*, *38*(3), 611–624. DOI: 10.1002/bin.1956

Williams, F., Gibbs, S., & Addo, A. S. (2022). The assessment and management of pica in people with intellectual disability. *BJPsych Advances*, *28*(6), 391–400. DOI: 10.1192/bja.2022.24

Willmott, E., Dickinson, R., Hall, C., Sadikovic, K., Wadhera, E., Micali, N., Trompeter, N., & Jewell, T. (2024). A scoping review of psychological interventions and outcomes for avoidant and restrictive food intake disorder (ARFID). *International Journal of Eating Disorders*, *57*(1), 27–61. DOI: 10.1002/eat.24073 PMID: 37876356

Zipfel, S., Giel, K. E., Bulik, C. M., Hay, P., & Schmidt, U. (2015). Anorexia nervosa: Aetiology, assessment, and treatment. *The Lancet. Psychiatry*, *2*(12), 1099–1111. https://www.thelancet.com/journals/lanpsy/article/PIIS2215-0366(15)00356-9/fulltext. DOI: 10.1016/S2215-0366(15)00356-9 PMID: 26514083

KEY TERMS AND DEFINITIONS

Behavioral Weight Loss Intervention: A program that helps people with binge-eating disorder to eat balanced meals and engage in moderate exercise, to reduce binging and promote physical health.

Cognitive Remediation Therapy (CRT): A treatment modality that helps improve flexibility and attention to change rigid thinking patterns.

Evidence-Based Practice: Refers to using treatment strategies that are based on research evidence and also align with client preferences and clinician expertise.

Guided Self-Help: Programs that provide people with workbooks or other structured tools to help them work through their treatment at their own pace.

Refeeding: A medical intervention that helps a person with severe malnutrition to gain weight.

Specialist Supportive Clinical Management (SSCM): A treatment strategy combining psychoeducation about eating disorders with supportive counseling.

Transcranial Direct Current Stimulation (tDCS): A non-invasive brain stimulation technique that may be effective for improving symptoms of anorexia nervosa.

Chapter 5
Cognitive Behavioral Therapy for Eating Disorders

ABSTRACT

This chapter explores the use of cognitive behavioral therapy (CBT), particularly enhanced CBT (CBT-E), in treating eating disorders. It outlines CBT's core principles, including the identification and restructuring of distorted thoughts and behaviors, and explains how CBT-E is adapted to address eating disorders like anorexia nervosa, bulimia nervosa, binge-eating disorder, and ARFID. The chapter describes the four stages of CBT-E and emphasizes its effectiveness across diverse populations. Case examples illustrate real-world applications, showing how CBT-E promotes recovery by targeting the psychological, behavioral, and emotional components of disordered eating.

INTRODUCTION

As indicated in the previous chapter, cognitive behavioral therapy (CBT) is often considered as the first line of treatment for eating disorders. Enhanced CBT is beneficial for treating adults with anorexia nervosa, and there is some evidence supporting this approach for adolescents (Brockmeyer et al., 2018). For bulimia nervosa, CBT specific to eating disorders is the most effective modality for achieving remission, according

DOI: 10.4018/979-8-3373-0664-3.ch005

to meta-analytic research (Hagan & Walsh, 2021; Slade et al., 2018). CBT is also effective for treating adolescents with bulimia nervosa (Hagan & Walsh, 2021; Hail & Le Grange, 2018). Finally, CBT is the gold standard for reducing binge-eating behaviors in binge-eating disorder (da Luz et al., 2020; Grilo, 2017; Hilbert et al., 2019), and it may be beneficial for treating some cases of ARFID and rumination disorder (Archibald & Bryant-Waugh, 2023; Sasegbon et al., 2022; Willmott et al., 2024).

Given the effectiveness and versatility of CBT approaches in eating disorder treatment, it is essential for clinicians to understand principles of CBT. The present chapter discusses the cognitive-behavioral approach, beginning with an overview of the modality and progressing to a discussion of CBT interventions adapted specifically for eating disorder treatment. The chapter concludes with several different case presentations, to demonstrate the application of CBT to the treatment of patients with eating disorders.

THE CBT TREATMENT MODALITY

Cognitive behavioral therapy (CBT) has roots in the work of Aaron Beck, who originally referred to his modality as cognitive therapy. Since its inception, numerous studies have found that CBT is effective for treating a range of psychiatric conditions, including anxiety, depression, bipolar disorder, schizophrenia, substance use disorders, personality disorders, and eating disorders. Beck developed the CBT modality after recognizing that many clients presenting with depression had distorted thinking patterns, and he posited that these distorted patterns are the cause of psychiatric problems. Distorted thinking patterns, also called cognitive distortions, are negative, biased ways of thinking, such as believing that everything is all good or all bad. People tend to become quite accustomed to acting on these cognitive distortions. As such, cognitive behavioral modalities emphasize automatic thoughts, which are immediate interpretations that lead to an emotional reaction, as well as cognitive distortions, such as believing the worst possible outcome will always occur, even when such an outcome is unlikely (Chand et al., 2023; Curtiss et al., 2021).

The ultimate goal of CBT is to replace distorted, unhelpful thoughts with new, more adaptive ways of thinking. The underlying belief in this modality is that when these thinking patterns change, emotions and behavior will follow suit, leading to improvements in functioning. A therapist who practices CBT works with clients to define their individual problems and develop goals for treatment. The therapist is likely to assign homework between sessions to help clients identify distorted thinking patterns and develop solutions for more adaptive ways of thinking about life events (Chand et al. 2023). During therapy sessions, a CBT clinician is likely to use cognitive restructuring, a technique that helps clients to consider alternative, more balanced ways of thinking (Curtiss et al., 2021).

Some CBT treatments incorporate other strategies, such as systematic desensitization, a type of exposure therapy that reduces anxiety by exposing a person to feared stimuli, beginning with stimuli that provoke lower levels of anxiety, and then moving up a hierarchy to include stimuli that provoke higher levels of anxiety. During exposure, a person practices calming strategies, such as muscle relaxation, so they learn to associate feared stimuli with calmness rather than distress (Thomas et al., 2017). Exposure therapy modalities are described in further detail in Chapter 8, which discusses other behavioral therapies, but they are worth mentioning here, as they may be incorporated into CBT treatment paradigms.

CBT IN EATING DISORDER TREATMENT

As previously mentioned, CBT is commonly used in eating disorder treatment, and it's considered an effective modality, based on research. Eating disorder professionals typically use an adapted version of CBT, called enhanced cognitive behavioral therapy (CBT-E), which is specific to eating disorders (Zipfel et al. 2015). In addition to using general CBT principles, the CBT-E modality addresses problems that are common in individuals with eating disorders, such as perfectionism, interpersonal conflict, low self-esteem, and difficulties with tolerating moods (Hagan & Walsh, 2021). CBT-E is divided into the following four stages (Zipfel et al., 2015):

- Stage one: Establishing mutual understanding between client and therapist of the client's eating disorder and working toward stabilizing eating patterns
- Stage two: Reviewing progress and planning for the main work of treatment
- Stage three: Addressing underlying beliefs related to body shape and eating that maintain eating disorder symptoms
- Stage four: Planning to manage future setbacks and sustain changes made during treatment

There is also a specific form of CBT developed for treating bulimia nervosa, formally called cognitive behavioral therapy for BN (CBT-BN). In CBT-BN, the underlying belief is that people diet because of concerns related to body weight and shape, which ultimately leads to binge eating, followed by inappropriate compensatory methods, such as self-induced vomiting or excessive exercise. As a person binges, their concerns related to body shape are reinforced, which perpetuates the cycle of dieting followed by binge-eating and purging. After helping a patient to normalize eating patterns, a therapist practicing CBT-BN works with the individual to restructure unhelpful thoughts related to body shape and weight (Hagan & Walsh, 2021).

Standard CBT approaches are utilized in patients with binge-eating disorder. Such approaches begin with the establishment of a collaborative relationship, as well as a phase of psychoeducation related to binge-eating disorder and principles of CBT. In the initial phase of treatment, patients also work with their therapist to identify unhealthy binge-eating patterns, primarily using self-monitoring approaches. During the middle phase of treatment, the focus shifts to the therapist and patient working together to challenge distorted thoughts related to weight, body shape, and stressors that trigger binge-eating. CBT treatment for binge-eating disorder concludes with planning for relapse prevention and maintaining healthy eating patterns (Grilo, 2017).

As with the other eating disorders, there are also CBT modalities specifically adapted for conditions like ARFID. Such modalities have been found to be helpful for both children and adults, as they can lead to the acceptance of new foods, as well as weight gain among patients who are underweight. CBT modalities used in ARFID treatment follow stages, as with other CBT treatments specific to eating disorders. ARFID-specific CBT models include psychoeducation, development of regular eating schedules, incorporation of new foods into the diet, education related to the risks of nutritional deficiencies, exposure to new foods, and relapse prevention planning (Thomas et al., 2021).

Potential Mechanisms Underlying the Benefits of CBT for Eating Disorders

Recent research highlights that the cognitive-behavioral model of eating disorders can be understood in relation to underlying neurobiological and cognitive processes. Individuals with eating disorders often show deficits in cognitive flexibility, or the ability to shift between different ways of thinking. For example, patients with anorexia nervosa frequently display rigid thinking styles, such as an extreme preoccupation with dietary rules or body image concerns. Neuroimaging studies suggest these rigid patterns are linked to dysfunction in neural circuits involving the prefrontal cortex and striatum, which are associated with goal-directed behavior and habit formation (Steward et al., 2017). CBT directly targets these rigid thought patterns by encouraging patients to generate alternative, more adaptive cognitions, thereby strengthening cognitive flexibility over time.

Another neurocognitive factor implicated in eating disorders is inhibitory control, or the ability to suppress automatic impulses. Deficits in inhibitory control have been observed in binge-eating disorder and bulimia nervosa, where urges to binge override long-term health goals. In research, individuals who binge-eat have been found to show reduced activation in areas of the prefrontal cortex, which is responsible for impulse control, when engaging in tasks that require them to override the desire to eat. This reduced activation may explain the difficulties with controlling food intake that occur with bulimia nervosa and binge-eating disorder (Berner et al., 2023). Furthermore, individuals with binge-eating disorder and bulimia nervosa may find food to be more rewarding than average, and approaches like CBT can be helpful for addressing both increased reward sensitivity and impaired inhibitory control. CBT strengthens inhibitory control by inserting a pause between cue and action, linking automatic thoughts to choices and long-term recovery goals (Pasquale et al., 2024).

CASE STUDIES

Now that a basic understanding of CBT modalities in eating disorder treatment has been established, it's helpful to gain exposure to case studies, to demonstrate this modality in action. Several case presentations are detailed below.

Case Presentation of CBT-E for Anorexia Nervosa

Jessica, a 23-year-old university student, presents to treatment with restrictive eating and significant weight loss, resulting in a BMI of 16.8, in line with diagnostic criteria for anorexia nervosa. She shows an intense fear of weight gain, as well as a distorted body image, perfectionistic tendencies, and strained family dynamics. Jessica's therapist, a licensed clinical social worker, works through the following stages of CBT-E with Jessica:

- **Stage 1:** Psychoeducation on nutritional rehabilitation and the impact of starvation on mental health. Jessica and her therapist collaboratively tracked food intake and worked on establishing regular meals/snacks.
- **Stage 2:** Evaluated Jessica's progress; identified that perfectionism and control were maintaining her restrictive behaviors.
- **Stage 3:** Challenged core beliefs such as "I must be thin to be successful." Behavioral experiments, such as eating feared foods and evaluating Jessica's reaction, were introduced.
- **Stage 4:** Planned for relapse prevention, explored how academic stressors could trigger relapse, and created coping strategies.

Over the course of the 16-week treatment program, Jessica gained 10 pounds and achieved a healthy BMI of 19.7. As a result of CBT interventions, her body image improved, and she began eating socially, rather than avoiding social outings at restaurants.

Case Presentation of CBT-E for Bulimia Nervosa

Carlos is a 17-year-old high school senior, who presented to treatment and reported that he is binge-eating three to four times per week, after which he forces himself to vomit. Carlos is extremely dissatisfied with his body and has withdrawn from his friends and family. Carlos sees a psychologist who specializes in the treatment of bulimia nervosa, and he collaborates with his psychologist through the following stages of CBT-E:

- **Stage 1:** Normalized eating patterns; Carlos kept a daily food and emotion log.
- **Stage 2:** Therapist identified that body-checking and fear of social judgment maintained binge-purge cycles.
- **Stage 3:** Used cognitive restructuring to challenge Carlos' belief of "If I'm not thin, no one will like me."
- **Stage 4:** Developed a safety plan for lapses during exam stress, identified peer supports.

After 12 weeks of treatment, Carlos reduced his binge-purge cycles to once per month. He was able to return to participating in sports, and he began feeling comfortable enough to eat lunch with his friends at school.

Case Presentation of CBT-E for ARFID

Stella is a 10-year-old child whose parents report she is an extremely picky eater. She will only consume five different foods, and she refuses all fruits, vegetables, and meats. Her parents have brought Stella to treatment because her eating habits have left her underweight with low energy levels. A pediatric psychologist progresses through the following stages of CBT-E with Stella's family:

- **Stage 1:** Discussed nutritional needs with Stella and her parents; introduced self-monitoring of food preferences.
- **Stage 2:** Built a hierarchy of "challenging foods." Introduced one new food weekly.

- **Stage 3:** Used systematic desensitization and reward-based reinforcement to encourage consumption of new foods.
- **Stage 4:** Educated family on relapse signs; created a home-based exposure plan for continued food trials.

After 20 weeks of CBT-E specific to ARFID, Stella accepted 20 new foods and gained weight, so she fell within the normal range for her age and height.

LIMITATIONS TO THE COGNITIVE-BEHAVIORAL APPROACH IN EATING DISORDER TREATMENT

Researchers have concluded that CBT, and particularly its enhanced version, is the gold standard for treating eating disorders, especially bulimia nervosa and binge-eating disorder. As such, this treatment modality should be included in the toolbox of all eating disorder therapists. Nonetheless, CBT is not without limitations. A significant portion of patients who undergo CBT do not achieve recovery; in fact, remission rates are only around 40%. This means over half of patients treated with CBT, which is the gold standard, will not reach remission. Furthermore, implementing the enhanced version of CBT can be time-consuming and expensive in community settings, so therapists may turn to modified formats. These modified versions can be effective, but there is limited research confirming their benefits (Agras & Bohon, 2021).

Based on the potential limitations of CBT, there is a need for additional research exploring methods for improving this modality, particularly with respect to remission rates. Furthermore, clinicians must understand that if they do not follow CBT exactly according to treatment protocols, they may not see the same benefits that occur in controlled trials using manualized CBT interventions specifically designed to treat eating disorders. Finally, it cannot be assumed that CBT will work for every patient with an eating disorder, despite its status as the first line of treatment. Sometimes, a clinician may need to use an alternative method with a particular client, or use additional interventions alongside CBT to promote symptom improvement.

CONCLUSION

As indicated in the case presentations above, CBT-E can be applied to the various different eating disorders, to help patients learn about their eating habits and overcome distorted or dysfunctional beliefs related to food and body image. General CBT principles, such as identifying and altering distorted thinking patterns, can be especially helpful for individuals with eating disorders. For instance, a patient with anorexia nervosa can identity distorted thoughts, such as the belief that her worth is entirely based on her body weight, and learn to replace such beliefs with healthier ways of thinking.

General CBT principles can be beneficial for changing distorted thinking patterns linked to eating disorder behaviors, but many successful CBT programs for eating disorders are adapted to be eating disorder-specific. For instance, CBT-E emphasizes problems related to eating disorders, helps patients to normalize eating patterns, and addresses negative beliefs related to weight and body shape using a stage-based model (Hagan & Walsh, 2021; Zipfel et al., 2015). Researchers and clinicians have also developed evidence-based models specific to certain eating disorders, including bulimia nervosa, binge-eating disorder, and ARFID (Grilo, 2017; Hagan & Walsh, 2021; Thomas et al., 2021). The bottom line is that CBT principles are applicable to the treatment of eating disorders, and they can be adapted to meet a client's unique case presentation. Nonetheless, clinicians must be aware of the potential limitations of CBT and prepared to adapt modalities to meet the needs of patients who do not improve with CBT (Agras & Bohon, 2021).

REFERENCES

Agras, W. S., & Bohon, C. (2021). Cognitive behavioral therapy for the eating disorders. *Annual Review of Clinical Psychology*, *17*(1), 417–438. DOI: 10.1146/annurev-clinpsy-081219-110907 PMID: 33962536

Archibald, T., & Bryant-Waugh, R. (2023). Current evidence for avoidant restrictive food intake disorder: Implications for clinical practice and future directions. *JCPP Advances*, *3*(2), e12160. DOI: 10.1002/jcv2.12160 PMID: 37753149

Berner, L. A., Winter, S. R., Ayaz, H., Shewokis, P. A., Izzetoglu, M., Marsh, R., Nasser, J. A., Matteucci, A. J., & Lowe, M. R. (2023). Altered prefrontal activation during the inhibition of eating responses in women with bulimia nervosa. *Psychological Medicine*, *53*(8), 3513–3523. DOI: 10.1017/S0033291722000198 PMID: 35209961

Brockmeyer, T., Friederich, H. C., & Schmidt, U. (2018). Advances in the treatment of anorexia nervosa: A review of established and emerging interventions. *Psychological Medicine*, *48*(8), 1228–1256. DOI: 10.1017/S0033291717002604 PMID: 28889819

Chand, S. P., Kuckel, D. P., & Huecker, M. R. (2023). Cognitive behavior therapy. In *StatPearls*. StatPearls Publishing., https://www.ncbi.nlm.nih.gov/books/NBK470241/

Curtiss, J. E., Levine, D. S., Ander, I., & Baker, A. W. (2021). Cognitive-behavioral treatments for anxiety and stress-related disorders. *Focus (San Francisco, Calif.)*, *19*(2), 142–149. DOI: 10.1176/appi.focus.20200045 PMID: 34690581

da Luz, F. Q., Hay, P., Wisniewski, L., Cordás, T., & Sainsbury, A. (2020). The treatment of binge eating disorder with cognitive behavior therapy and other therapies: An overview and clinical considerations. *Obesity Reviews*, *22*(5, S1), e13180. DOI: 10.1111/obr.13180 PMID: 33350574

Grilo, C. M. (2017). Psychological and behavioral treatments for binge-eating disorder. *The Journal of Clinical Psychiatry*, *78*(Suppl 1), 20–24. DOI: 10.4088/JCP.sh16003su1c.04 PMID: 28125175

Hagan, K. E., & Walsh, B. T. (2021). State of the art: The therapeutic approaches to bulimia nervosa. *Clinical Therapeutics*, *43*(1), 40–49. DOI: 10.1016/j.clinthera.2020.10.012 PMID: 33358256

Hail, L., & Le Grange, D. (2018). Bulimia nervosa in adolescents: Prevalence and treatment challenges. *Adolescent Health, Medicine and Therapeutics*, *9*, 11–16. DOI: 10.2147/AHMT.S135326 PMID: 29379324

Hilbert, A., Petroff, D., Herpertz, S., Pietrowsky, R., Tuschen-Caffier, B., Vocks, S., & Schmidt, R. (2019). Meta-analysis of the efficacy of psychological and medical treatments for binge-eating disorder. *Journal of Consulting and Clinical Psychology*, *87*(1), 91–105. DOI: 10.1037/ccp0000358 PMID: 30570304

Pasquale, E. K., Boyar, A. M., & Boutelle, K. N. (2024). Reward and inhibitory control as mechanisms and treatment targets for binge eating disorder. *Current Psychiatry Reports*, *26*(9), 616–625. DOI: 10.1007/s11920-024-01534-z PMID: 39316228

Sasegbon, A., Hasan, S. S., Disney, B. R., & Vasant, D. H. (2022). Rumination syndrome: Pathophysiology, diagnosis and practical management. *Frontline Gastroenterology*, *13*(5), 402–409. DOI: 10.1136/flgastro-2021-101856 PMID: 36046491

Slade, E., Keeney, E., Mavranezouli, I., Dias, S., Fou, L., Stockton, S., Saxon, L., Waller, G., Turner, H., Serpell, L., Fairburn, C. G., & Kendall, T. (2018). Treatments for bulimia nervosa: A network meta-analysis. *Psychological Medicine*, *48*(16), 2629–2636. DOI: 10.1017/S0033291718001071 PMID: 29729686

Steward, T., Menchón, J. M., Jiménez-Murcia, S., Soriano-Mas, C., & Fernández-Aranda, F. (2017). Neural network alterations across eating disorders: A narrative review of fMRI studies. *Current Neuropharmacology*, *15*(5), 1–13. DOI: 10.2174/1570159X15666171017111532 PMID: 29046154

Thomas, J. J., Becker, K. R., Breithaupt, L., Burton Murray, H., Jo, J. H., Kuhnle, M. C., Dreier, M. J., Harshman, S., Kahn, D. L., Hauser, K., Slattery, M., Misra, M., Lawson, E. A., & Eddy, K. T. (2021). Cognitive-behavioral therapy for adults with avoidant/restrictive food intake disorder. *Journal of Behavioral and Cognitive Therapy*, *31*(1), 47–55. DOI: 10.1016/j.jbct.2020.10.004 PMID: 34423319

Thomas, K., Dowd, C., & Broman-Fulks, J. J. (2017). Systematic desensitization. In Zeigler-Hill, V., & Shackelford, T. K. (Eds.), *Encyclopedia of personality and individual differences* (pp. 1–3). Springer., DOI: 10.1007/978-3-319-28099-8_952-1

Willmott, E., Dickinson, R., Hall, C., Sadikovic, K., Wadhera, E., Micali, N., Trompeter, N., & Jewell, T. (2024). A scoping review of psychological interventions and outcomes for avoidant and restrictive food intake disorder (ARFID). *International Journal of Eating Disorders*, *57*(1), 27–61. DOI: 10.1002/eat.24073 PMID: 37876356

Zipfel, S., Giel, K. E., Bulik, C. M., Hay, P., & Schmidt, U. (2015). Anorexia nervosa: Aetiology, assessment, and treatment. *The Lancet. Psychiatry*, *2*(12), 1099–1111. https://www.thelancet.com/journals/lanpsy/article/PIIS2215-0366(15)00356-9/fulltext. DOI: 10.1016/S2215-0366(15)00356-9 PMID: 26514083

KEY TERMS AND DEFINITIONS

Automatic Thoughts: Immediate interpretations of events, which tend to be negative and lead to an emotional reaction

Cognitive Behavioral Therapy (CBT): A treatment modality that aims to replace distorted thinking patterns with new, healthier ways of thinking, to alleviate distress and promote desired behavioral change

Cognitive Behavioral Therapy for BN (CBT-BN): A version of CBT adapted for use with patients with bulimia nervosa, based on the underlying belief that concerns related to body shape lead people to diet, which in turn leads to binging and purging

Cognitive Distortions: Biased, negative thinking patterns that tend to lead to distress

Cognitive Restructuring: A process in CBT that aims to help clients consider alternative, more balanced explanations for situations, to reduce their anxiety

Cognitive Therapy: Aaron Beck's original model, which formed the foundation for CBT

Enhanced Cognitive Behavioral Therapy (CBT-E): A specific form of CBT adapted for use in patients with eating disorders

CASE NOTES

Case Presentation of CBT-E for Anorexia Nervosa

Questions

1. What symptoms of anorexia nervosa does Jessica display?
2. What evidence of distorted thinking does Jessica display?
3. How could the therapist use cognitive restructuring with Jessica?
4. Can treatment with CBT-E be considered successful?
5. What additional intervention might you recommend for Jessica?

Epilogue and Lessons Learned

Jessica displays symptoms of anorexia nervosa, including low BMI, intense fear of weight gain, and body image distortion. She shows evidence of distorted thinking, as she believes she must be thin to be successful. The therapist could use cognitive restructuring by helping Jessica to explore alternative indicators of success, such as athletic accomplishments, specific skills she possesses, academic achievements, or personality traits, such as kindness. CBT-E appears to have been successful for Jessica, as she is restored to a healthy weight, based on BMI. Given that she experiences family strain, Jessica may also benefit from family-based interventions.

Case Presentation of CBT-E for Bulimia Nervosa

Questions

1. What symptoms of bulimia nervosa does Carlos show?
2. How do we know his symptoms aren't better explained by binge-eating disorder?
3. What evidence of cognitive distortion does Carlos display?
4. What would Carlos' therapist explore with him when engaging in cognitive restructuring?
5. What evidence of treatment success is present in Carlos' case?

Epilogue and Lessons Learned

Carlos shows symptoms of bulimia nervosa, including repeated episodes of binge-eating, forced vomiting, and body dissatisfaction. He does not meet criteria for binge-eating disorder, as he is using the inappropriate compensatory strategy of forced vomiting; binge-eating disorder does not involve inappropriate compensatory strategies. Carlos displays evidence of cognitive distortions, because he states that no one will like him if he isn't thin. Carlos' therapist could explore evidence against this thought in cognitive restructuring. For instance, she could ask for evidence of things people like about Carlos that have nothing to do with his weight or body size. Carlos shows evidence of treatment success, based on reduced episodes of binging and purging and improved functioning (ie: participating in sports and eating lunch with friends).

Case Presentation of CBT-E for ARFID

Questions

1. What diagnostic criteria does Stella demonstrate for ARFID?
2. How do we know that Stella's symptoms aren't better-explained by anorexia nervosa?
3. What cognitive distortions might Stella have that perpetuate her symptoms?
4. How could cognitive restructuring be added to Stella's treatment?
5. Can Stella's treatment be considered a success?

Epilogue and Lessons Learned

Stella demonstrates diagnostic criteria for ARFID, including food refusal, and showing failure to grow (ie: low body weight) due to her food refusal. While Stella is underweight, her symptoms are not better-explained by anorexia nervosa, because there is no indication in her case presentation that she has a body image disturbance or that she is restricting food due to fear of weight gain. Instead, she is a picky eater, who refuses foods based on her pickiness. This aligns better with ARFID. Based on her ARFID diagnosis, Stella may believe that she will experience intense displeasure or becoming seriously ill if she tries a new food. Based on this distortion, the therapist could use cognitive restructuring to help Stella identify alternative outcomes that may occur when trying new foods, which could include liking the new foods, having a neutral opinion toward them, or simply disliking them and moving on without serious side effects. Ultimately, Stella's treatment appears successful, as she gained weight and tried a significant number of new foods.

List of Additional Sources (for all case presentations in this chapter)

The following readings are beneficial for behavioral health clinicians and clinicians-in-training who are seeking to learn more about CBT, and specifically, its applications in eating disorder treatment:

1. Beck, J.S. (2020). *Cognitive behavioral therapy: Basics and beyond.* The Guilford Press.
2. Dalle Grave, R., & Calugi, S. (2020). *Cognitive behavior therapy for adolescents with eating disorders.* The Guilford Press.
3. Fairburn, C.G. (2008). *Cognitive behavior therapy and eating disorders.* The Guilford Press.

Chapter 6
Dialectical Behavior Therapy for Eating Disorders

ABSTRACT

This chapter explores the application of Dialectical Behavior Therapy (DBT) to eating disorders, tracing its evolution from a treatment for suicidal behaviors to an evidence-based approach for emotional dysregulation and maladaptive coping. It outlines DBT's theoretical foundations, including dialectics, biosocial theory, and behavioral principles. The chapter details DBT's four treatment stages, core skills modules, and service delivery components. Adaptations such as the Stanford model for bulimia nervosa and binge-eating disorder and RO-DBT for anorexia nervosa are discussed. Case studies illustrate DBT's effectiveness in reducing disordered eating behaviors and improving emotion regulation.

INTRODUCTION

Dialectical behavior therapy (DBT) has origins in behavioral theory, but given its distinctiveness as a therapeutic modality, it warrants its own chapter. Masha Linehan is credited with the development of DBT, which she originally designed for treating individuals with extreme suicidal behaviors. While DBT was developed to meet the needs of those with suicidal behavior, it eventually expanded to become an evidence-based

DOI: 10.4018/979-8-3373-0664-3.ch006

treatment for borderline personality disorder (BPD). DBT originally emphasized the teaching of problem-solving skills, but many patients rejected this focus, viewing it as invalidating. In response, Linehan adjusted the DBT modality to emphasize a balance of change and acceptance, which is what this modality continues to be known for today. In its early stages, DBT focused on meeting the needs of individuals with BPD, many of whom had co-occurring disorders, such as depression, anxiety, and eating disorders (Linehan & Wilks, 2015). Today, DBT is used in the treatment of a variety of different disorders, including eating disorders (Brown et al., 2020). The current chapter discusses the DBT modality, beginning with a general overview and then progressing to in-depth discussion of the use of DBT in eating disorder treatment.

CORE ASSUMPTIONS OF THE DBT MODALITY

The foundational assumption underlying DBT is the centrality of dialectics, which refers to the coming together of opposing ideas. In DBT, the main dialectic is between acceptance and change. On the one hand, a patient must learn to tolerate their own distress, while also receiving validation from an accepting therapist. On the other hand, the therapist must guide the client toward changing unhelpful behaviors (Linehan & Wilks 2015). In DBT, the concept of dialectics doesn't just apply to the tension between acceptance and change; it is present throughout all facets of treatment. For instance, a patient participating in DBT is likely to learn that it's possible to hold two opposing views at once, and there may be some truth in both views. The tension between two opposing views can also be the very thing that brings about change in a patient. Ultimately, DBT teaches patients to tolerate reality and accept themselves, while also teaching them the skills necessary for making desired behavioral changes (Rizvi et al., 2013).

Also foundational to the DBT model is the biosocial theory, which argues that emotion dysregulation, a core symptom of BPD and other disorders, is the result of the interaction between biological sensitivities and an unsupportive environment. Biological sensitivities cause the body's emotion regulation system to operate in a dysfunctional manner, causing emotional sensitivity, overreactivity, and a slow return to baseline after experiencing an intense emotion. When these sensitivities are paired with an environment in which one's emotions are not honored, a person may have to express themselves in an intense fashion. For instance, a child whose parents do not honor their need for security may scream, cry, and throw tantrums to obtain attention. Furthermore, an environment that fails to validate one's emotions is also likely to neglect to teach a child proper emotion regulation skills. Such an environment teaches a person they must express themselves intensely when communicating an emotional need, while leaving them without the skills needed to regulate their own emotions (Rizvi et al., 2013).

Finally, DBT is rooted in behavioral theory, so this treatment modality emphasizes interventions that help a person to reduce their engagement in maladaptive behaviors while increasing their use of adaptive behaviors. As a behaviorally-oriented therapy, DBT evaluates unhelpful behavior in terms of antecedents (what occurs before the behavior) and consequences (what occurs in response to the behavior). In alignment with behavioral theory, the DBT modality also posits that unhelpful behaviors occur because of lack of skill, cognitive factors, emotional processing deficiencies, and reinforcements. (Rizvi et al., 2013). Alongside biosocial theory and the concept of dialectics, behavioral theory informs DBT-based treatments.

COMPONENTS OF DBT TREATMENT

The aforementioned theoretical foundation guides the DBT modality, which involves four stages of treatment as well as the teaching of specific skills. In the first stage of treatment, the therapist works towards stabilizing the patient and helping the pain to gain control over life-threatening behaviors like suicide attempts and self-injurious acts. This initial stage also aims to reduce the occurrence of behaviors that impede progress in therapy. These behaviors include missing appointments and refusal to engage in the treatment process. Once a patient has been stabilized, they can proceed to stage two, in which they have learned to control harmful behaviors, but emotional pain remains. During the second stage, patients must allow themselves to experience their emotions and process any unresolved trauma. Stage three aims to address routine problems of living, and during stage four, the client arrives at a sense of completeness and finds joy in life (Linehan & Wilks, 2015). Beyond this stage model of treatment, DBT involves a range of services as well as training in specific skills; these features of treatment are described in further detail in the sections that follow.

Not all patients participating in DBT progress through treatment in a linear fashion. A patient may progress to stage two, and then later regress to dangerous behaviors, placing the patient back in stage one. Diary cards are particularly useful in stage one of DBT; these cards allow patients to monitor their emotions, behaviors, and use of coping skills daily. The most severe behaviors or emotions noted on the diary card become the focus of the therapy session during stage one. For example, if diary cards indicate the presence of suicidal behavior, overcoming this behavior is the focus of the session. In some cases, behaviors during stage one might be less severe, involving tendencies like showing up late to appointments or using substances. Regardless of the specific focus of the session, the therapist works with the patient to determine events, thoughts, and feelings that contributed to the problem behavior and to identify consequences of the behavior. Then, therapist and patient collaborate to identify how the chain of events leading to the problem behavior could be broken. This may involve role-playing during sessions to practice interrupting the chain (Rizvi et al., 2013).

SERVICES PROVIDED IN DBT

DBT services center on four treatment modes: individual therapy, group skills training, consultation with the therapist between sessions, and therapist team meetings. In addition to participating in individual therapy, patients in DBT treatment attend group skills training sessions. The purpose of skills training sessions is to teach patients new behaviors that can take the place of maladaptive behaviors. Skills training includes the following four modules: mindfulness, interpersonal effectiveness, emotion regulation, and distress tolerance. These skills are taught during group sessions, using strategies such as handouts, worksheets, story-telling, modeling, coaching, and rehearsal (Linehan & Wilks, 2015).

The four DBT skills can be defined as follows (Linehan & Wilks, 2015):

- **Mindfulness:** Core skills in DBT treatment that involve nonjudgmental awareness of the present, which includes being able to simply describe and observe emotions and experiences
- **Emotion regulation:** A set of skills, such as being able to identify emotions and manage painful feelings, which reduces undesirable emotional responses
- **Interpersonal effectiveness**: Skills that allow a person to more effectively address conflict with others and assert themselves
- **Distress tolerance:** The ability to accept, make meaning of, and cope with distress through self-soothing and delay of gratification

Outside of therapy and group skills training sessions, patients have access to their therapist via phone coaching, which occurs as needed to help patients use skills in daily life. The purpose of these phone coaching sessions is to help patients use their DBT skills; the intent is not to reinforce unhealthy coping mechanisms through therapist attention. Finally, therapists participate in a consultation team while providing DBT services in order to enhance their ability to provide treatment and to give them access to support and feedback (Rizvi et al., 2013).

DBT IN EATING DISORDER TREATMENT

DBT, with its focus on reducing problem behaviors and addressing emotion dysregulation, can be effective in the treatment of eating disorders. The behaviors associated with the eating disorders can be characterized as maladaptive methods for regulating emotions. In patients with binge-eating disorder, for instance, unpleasant emotions can trigger a binge-eating episode, during which food serves as a source of comfort (Bankoff et al., 2012).

Consider also the biosocial theory underlying DBT, which posits that emotion regulation difficulties occur due to the interaction between emotional vulnerabilities and an unsupportive environment (Rizvi et al., 2013). This theory can be applied to eating disorders, which may occur in individuals who not only experience emotional sensitivities but who also show difficulty identifying hunger and satiety cues. These sensitivities can occur in both unsupportive family environments and within the larger cultural context, which tends to stigmatize larger bodies (Bankoff et al., 2012). So, eating disorders can be conceptualized in a way that aligns with the core assumptions of the DBT model.

An older research review, conducted by Bankoff et al. (2012), revealed that treatments based on DBT were effective for reducing eating disorder symptoms and improving mood. Most studies included in the review found that DBT was effective for reducing binge-eating, purging, and food restriction. The review also found that DBT was effective for reducing self–injury and suicidal behavior, as well as for preventing treatment dropout and treating co-occurring disorders. While the studies in the review did not directly measure emotion regulation, the underlying belief in many of the studies was that emotion regulation is the most important component of DBT for eating disorders (Bankoff et al., 2012). This belief prevails in the eating disorder treatment realm, with anorexia nervosa conceptualized as a disorder of emotional overcontrol, while bulimia nervosa and binge-eating disorder are characterized as disorders of emotional undercontrol. Both ends of the spectrum involve the use of eating disorder behaviors to attempt to regulate emotional states (Ben-Porath et al, 2020).

A more recent research review also revealed beneficial effects of DBT for eating disorders. More specifically, DBT has been found to reduce the occurrence of binge-eating in those with binge-eating disorder. It has also been found to lead to decreases in body weight and improvements in emotional regulation skills for those with binge-eating disorder. There are specific DBT modalities adapted for the treatment of eating disorders. For example, the Stanford model is used to treat both binge-eating disorder and bulimia nervosa; it views binge-eating and purging as maladaptive ways to regulate painful emotions. Therefore, the focus of the model is addressing deficits in emotion regulation. This model has been found effective for reducing binge-eating in both bulimia nervosa and binge-eating disorder (Ben-Porath et al., 2020).

The Stanford model is not the only DBT adaptation designed for eating disorder treatment. The radically open DBT model (RO-DBT) has been adapted for the treatment of anorexia nervosa. According to this model, individuals with anorexia nervosa feel unsafe, because of their sensitivity to threat, combined with feedback from the environment. Food restriction serves as a way to weaken the effect of negative emotions in those with anorexia nervosa, according to RO-DBT models. This model also addresses the emotional overcontrol and cognitive rigidity that tend to occur in those with anorexia nervosa by teaching radical openness, which emphasizes flexibility and social connectedness. While this treatment does not directly promote weight gain, one study found that it led to significant weight gain in 72% of patients completing a treatment program (Ben-Porath et al., 2020).

CASE STUDIES

To fully understand the application of DBT in eating disorder treatment, it's helpful to review case studies using this modality. Below are three case studies, demonstrating how DBT interventions are applied to the treatment of eating disorders.

Case Study of DBT for Anorexia Nervosa (RO-DBT Model)

Lucía is a 29-year-old practicing attorney, who identifies as a perfectionist. She works long hours and pressures herself to submit flawless legal documentation. When Lucía makes small mistakes, she is harshly critical of herself and convinces herself she must work longer hours to avoid mistakes. During her assessment, Lucía reports that she likes to be in control. She counts every calorie and is extremely fearful of gaining weight and being seen as "sloppy" or "lazy." When she enters treatment, Lucía's BMI is dangerously low. Based on her apparent emotional undercontrol, Lucía's therapist determines that radically open DBT (RO-DBT) should be carried out, as follows:

- Lucía's therapist introduces her to RO-DBT to help Lucía overcome her emotional control and rigid thinking patterns. During early sessions, Lucia learns to practice radical openness and move away from her perfectionistic tendencies. Lucía learns to practice mindfulness and distress tolerance to help her cope with her urges to restrict food and attempt to control her environment.
- After 20 weeks of treatment, Lucía is able to increase her calorie intake, which helps her gain weight. She has increased her expression of emotions during therapy sessions, and she has reduced anxiety around eating. This progress demonstrates that Lucía has reduced her emotional overcontrol.

Case Study of DBT for Bulimia Nervosa (Stanford Model)

Jordan is a 26-year-old marketing professional seeking treatment for eating-related concerns. He reports that around twice per week, he experiences eating episodes during which he consumes such large amounts of food that he feels sick afterward. Despite knowing he will become sick from consuming such large quantities of food, Jordan is unable to control the amount of food he eats during these binges. Afterward, he feels incredibly ashamed of himself and immediately spends up to four hours jogging around his neighborhood to rid himself of the extra calories. After identifying that Jordan has a history of invalidating family dynamics and poor emotion regulation, his therapist decides to follow the Stanford Model of DBT, as described below:

- Jordan's therapist works with him to help him address deficits in emotion regulation. Throughout the course of therapy, Jordan is able to identify that his binge episodes often occur in response to interpersonal distress with his colleagues at work. Jordan attends individual DBT sessions and uses a diary card to track his emotions and behaviors. This helps him to identify that interpersonal distress is typically the antecedent to his binge-eating episodes. Jordan also participates in DBT skills training groups, where he learns skills for tolerating stress from interactions with colleagues. Jordan learns to use self-soothing strategies or distraction when he is distressed and tempted to binge-eat.

- Jordan makes significant progress over the course of treatment. After 6 months, Jordan is only binge-eating and purging once monthly. He is able to identify his emotional triggers and apply emotion regulation strategies when feeling triggered. This allows him to gain better control over his impulsive urges to binge-eat.

Case Study of DBT for Binge-Eating Disorder

Marquell is a 38-year-old school counselor who comes to treatment for assistance managing repeated episodes of binge-eating. He tends to binge-eat right after getting home from work in the late afternoon. Marquell describes feelings of being numb and overwhelmed during these binge-eating episodes. He sometimes consumes half of a week's worth of groceries during these episodes, leading him to feel guilty and ashamed afterward. Marquell's therapist operates according to the biosocial model, and he identifies both emotional sensitivities and an invalidating family environment during childhood as contributing to Marquell's struggles. Given this fact, the therapist employs the following DBT treatment modality for Marquell:

- Marquell participates in individual sessions with his therapist to process the skills he is learning in a DBT skills group. Marquell's therapist also teaches him to use diary cards so he can track how he is feeling before a binge. During group sessions, Marquell learns to use mindfulness skills to help him identify his emotional states prior to a binge. He also learns distress tolerance strategies, such as splashing cold water on his face or using deep breathing to manage intense emotions.
- By week 12 of treatment, Marquell has almost completely eliminated his binge-eating episodes. Using diary cards has helped him to link uncomfortable emotions to his eating behaviors. Group skills

training sessions have also helped him develop coping skills that do not involve binge-eating.

LIMITATIONS OF DBT IN EATING DISORDER TREATMENT

While DBT certainly has a role in eating disorder treatment, it is not without flaws. For example, DBT is an intensive treatment, and some organizations may have difficulty implementing a DBT program, so it may be difficult for patients to find a therapist who offers this type of service. It may be possible for a patient to locate a therapist who utilizes some features of the DBT modality, but who does not adhere exactly to DBT standards. Without complete fidelity to the DBT model, effectiveness may be reduced in actual treatment settings, as compared to in research (Carmel et al., 2014).

Finally, DBT is a time-consuming modality. Patients may find the combination of therapy and skills groups to be cumbersome. As such, this modality is not likely to be ideal for patients who have busy schedules or other commitments, such as work or parenting obligations. Offering DBT to patients is also time-consuming for clinicians, who may not be able to take on large caseloads. This further reduces access to DBT services (Carmel et al., 2014).

CONCLUSION

DBT, through its teaching of emotion regulation, distress tolerance, and mindfulness skills (Linehan & Wilks, 2015), can be beneficial for patients living with eating disorder symptoms. Since eating disorder symptoms can reflect poor emotion regulation skills, the core components of DBT can be effective for treating symptoms of disordered eating. Specific modalities have been adapted to meet the unique needs of patients with eating disorders (Bankoff et al., 2012; Ben-Porath et al., 2020). For patients whose eating disorder symptoms appear to be rooted in emotion dysregulation and poor distress tolerance, DBT can be the treatment modality of choice.

REFERENCES

Bankoff, S. M., Karpel, M. G., Forbes, H. E., & Pantalone, D. W. (2012). A systematic review of dialectical behavior therapy for the treatment of eating disorders. *Eating Disorders*, *20*(3), 196–215. DOI: 10.1080/10640266.2012.668478 PMID: 22519897

Ben-Porath, D., Duthu, F., Luo, T., Gonidakis, F., Compte, E. J., & Wisniewski, L. (2020). Dialectical behavior therapy: An update and review of the existing treatment models adapted for adults with eating disorders. *Eating Disorders*, *28*(2), 101–121. DOI: 10.1080/10640266.2020.1723371 PMID: 32129724

Brown, T. A., Wisniewski, L., & Anderson, L. K. (2020). Dialectical behavior therapy for eating disorders: State of the research and new directions. *Eating Disorders*, *28*(2), 97–100. DOI: 10.1080/10640266.2020.1728204 PMID: 32301685

Carmel, A., Rose, M., & Fruzzetti, A. E. (2014). Barriers and solutions to implementing dialectical behavior therapy in a public behavioral health system. *Administration and Policy in Mental Health*, *41*(5), 608–614. DOI: 10.1007/s10488-013-0504-6 PMID: 23754686

Linehan, M. M., & Wilks, C. R. (2015). The course and evolution of dialectical behavior therapy. *American Journal of Psychotherapy*, *69*(2), 97–110. DOI: 10.1176/appi.psychotherapy.2015.69.2.97 PMID: 26160617

Rizvi, S. L., Steffel, L. M., & Carson-Wong, A. (2013). An overview of dialectical behavior therapy for professional psychologists. *Professional Psychology, Research and Practice*, *44*(2), 73–80. DOI: 10.1037/a0029808

KEY TERMS AND DEFINITIONS

Biosocial theory: A foundation model in dialectical behavior therapy, which asserts that emotion regulation difficulties occur because of the interaction between biological sensitivities and invalidating environments

Dialectical Behavior Therapy (DBT): An intervention developed by Marsha Linehan that emphasizes learning skills related to mindfulness, emotion regulation, distress tolerance, and interpersonal effectiveness

Distress tolerance: A DBT skill that involves accepting and coping with distress by using self-soothing techniques and delay of gratification

Emotion regulation: A set of DBT skills that help a person identify emotions and manage painful feelings without engaging in undesirable emotional responses

Interpersonal effectiveness: DBT skills geared toward helping people manage conflict effectively and use assertiveness skills

Mindfulness: Core DBT skills that include nonjudgmental, present-moment awareness

Radically Open DBT (RO-DBT): A specific DBT model adapted for the treatment of anorexia nervosa, emphasizing radical openness to overcome emotional overcontrol

Stanford Model: A specific DBT model adapted for the treatment of bulimia nervosa and binge-eating disorder

CASE NOTES

Case Study of DBT for Anorexia Nervosa (RO-DBT Model)

Questions

1. What symptoms of anorexia nervosa does Lucía show?
2. What evidence do we have that Lucía's symptoms are linked to emotional dysregulation?
3. What features of DBT are present in Lucía's treatment?
4. As her therapist, what distress tolerance strategies might you recommend for Lucía?
5. What would it look like for Lucía to practice mindfulness?

Epilogue and Lessons Learned

Lucía shows symptoms of anorexia nervosa, including intense fear of weight gain and low BMI. These symptoms appear to be linked to a specific form of emotion dysregulation called emotional overcontrol. This is evident, based on Lucía showing a strong need for control and expecting perfection from herself. We see evidence of core DBT skills in Lucía's treatment, including learning mindfulness and distress tolerance. Some helpful distress tolerance strategies for Lucía might include distracting herself with a book or funny movie, or soothing herself through taking a warm bath or listening to calm music. For Lucía, practicing mindfulness would involve learning to recognize and simply observe painful emotions, such as shame, rather than suppressing these emotions and coping through food restriction.

Case Study of DBT for Bulimia Nervosa (Stanford Model)

Questions

1. What symptoms of bulimia nervosa does Jordan show?
2. Does Jordan meet the diagnostic threshold for frequency of symptoms?
3. How do we see evidence of biosocial theory in Jordan's case?
4. What core features of DBT are present in Jordan's case?
5. How do we see evidence of behavioral theory at play in Jordan's case?

Epilogue and Lessons Learned

Jordan shows symptoms of bulimia nervosa, including binge-eating, losing control while eating, and then ridding the body of excess calories via excessive exercise. These episodes occur twice per week, which meets the threshold of one episode per week, which is required for diagnosis. Jordan's case shows evidence of biosocial theory, because his symptoms are determined to be the result of invalidating family dynamics and poor emotion regulation skills. Biosocial theory would argue that Jordan's poor emotion regulation skills are due to some sort of biological sensitivity as well. We see several core features of DBT in Jordan's case, including participation in skills groups, the learning of distress tolerance skills, and the use of emotion regulation strategies. We also see evidence of behavioral theory at play, since Jordan is using diary cards to identify antecedents to problematic behaviors like binge-eating.

Case Study of DBT for Binge-Eating Disorder

Questions

1. What symptoms of binge-eating disorder does Marquell show?
2. Why would Marquell not qualify for a diagnosis of bulimia nervosa?
3. What features of DBT are present in Marquell's treatment?
4. What evidence do we have that DBT is an appropriate treatment for Marquell?
5. There is evidence of the biosocial model at play in Marquell's case; what other theory is at play?

Epilogue and Lessons Learned

Marquell shows symptoms of binge-eating disorder, including repeated episodes of binge-eating, followed by shame and guilt. He would not qualify for a diagnosis of bulimia nervosa, since there is no evidence of purging following binges. Marquell's treatment shows several features associated with DBT, including attending a DBT skills group and learning distress tolerance and mindfulness skills. DBT appears to be an appropriate treatment for Marquell, because his binge-eating episodes are linked to uncomfortable emotions. This would suggest that he is using binging as a maladaptive strategy for regulating emotions. Aside from the biosocial model, Marquell's case shows evidence of behavioral theory, since Marquell is using diary cards to identify emotional antecedents to binge-eating.

List of Additional Sources (for all case presentations in this chapter)

1. Chapman, A. L., & Dixon-Gordon, K. L. (2020). *Dialectical behavior therapy*. American Psychological Association. https://doi.org/10.1037/0000207-001

2. Safer, D. L., Telch, C. F., & Chen, E. Y. (2017). *Dialectical behavior therapy for binge eating and bulimia* (2nd ed.). Guilford Press.
3. Wisniewski, L., & Ben-Porath, D. D. (2015). Dialectical behavior therapy and eating disorders: The use of contingency management procedures to manage dialectical dilemmas. *American Journal of Psychotherapy, 69*(2), 129–142. https://doi.org/10.1176/appi.psychotherapy.2015.69.2.129

Chapter 7
Psychodynamic Therapy for Eating Disorders

ABSTRACT

This chapter explores the application of psychodynamic therapy in the treatment of eating disorders. Grounded in psychoanalytic theory, psychodynamic therapy emphasizes unconscious conflict, early attachment disruptions, and internalized relational patterns as key contributors to disordered eating. The chapter reviews foundational concepts such as defense mechanisms, transference, and the therapeutic alliance, and introduces contemporary extensions including object relations theory and self psychology. Psychodynamic conceptualizations of each major eating disorder are discussed, highlighting how disordered eating behaviors often serve as symbolic expressions of unmet emotional needs or unresolved trauma. Treatment strategies focus on gaining insight into internal dynamics, strengthening the sense of self, and resolving early relational wounds. Two case studies—one for anorexia nervosa and one for binge-eating disorder—illustrate how psychodynamic principles are applied in clinical settings.

INTRODUCTION

Given the history of eating disorder conceptualization and treatment, it is essential to consider psychodynamic modalities for treating patients with eating disorders. After all, experts began applying the psychoanalytic

DOI 10.4018/979-8-3373-0664-3.ch007

perspective to eating disorder treatment in the late 19th and early 20th centuries, recognizing that psychological factors contributed to eating disorders (Farrell, 1995). Today, therapeutic modalities derived from the psychoanalytic perspective show promise for alleviating eating disorder symptoms. While additional research is needed to determine the specific factors that lead to treatment success, a recent research review found that psychodynamic interventions were beneficial for treating eating disorders, especially anorexia nervosa (Abbate-Daga et al., 2016). The current chapter describes psychodynamic approaches to eating disorder treatment, beginning with a review of the theoretical underpinnings of these interventions, before describing their applications in eating disorder treatment.

CORE CONCEPTS IN PSYCHODYNAMIC THERAPY

Psychodynamic therapy has evolved from Sigmund Freud's psychoanalytic theory, which emphasized the role of unconscious drives, internal conflict, and early childhood experiences in shaping behavior. Freud's structural model of the psyche (id, ego, superego) and his focus on repression, dream analysis, and free association have influenced the development of psychodynamic approaches (Gabbard, 2004). While the terms psychodynamic and psychoanalytic are often used interchangeably, a more nuanced understanding of this modality recognizes that psychoanalysis refers to Freud's original theory, whereas the psychodynamic modality encompasses more modern approaches based on Freud's original ideas (Opland & Torrico, 2025). Nonetheless, both Freud's version of psychoanalysis, as well as current psychodynamic approaches, can play a role in effective eating disorder treatments.

Freud's original psychoanalytic theory emphasized the role of instinctual, unconscious drives, often sexual or aggressive in nature. According to Freud, people may experience psychological symptoms as they attempt to satisfy these instinctual drives. Freud further posited that because some mental conflicts are too painful for people to face, they suppress them into the subconscious mind, causing inexplicable emotional side effects. Also essential to understanding Freud's psychoanalytic theory is his division of human personality into three distinct states: the id, which is impulsive and seeks gratification; the ego, which is grounded in reality; and the superego, which contains the conscience, experiences guilt and drives a person to engage in moral behavior (Sue et al., 2017).

According to Freud, some internal conflicts are so painful that people cannot face them. To manage the anxiety associated with these internal conflicts, Freud asserted that people utilize defense mechanisms to protect themselves from facing unpleasant internal material. These defense mechanisms operate at the unconscious level, meaning that people are not cognizant of their use of these defenses. The ultimate goal of psychoanalytic therapy, then, is to help clients overcome these defenses by bringing unconscious material into the conscious mind, thereby allowing them to gain insight into their thoughts and unresolved childhood conflicts. Freud believed that this therapeutic goal could be achieved through free association, a process in which the client says whatever comes to mind during therapy, or through dream analysis, which, as the name might suggest, involves interpretation of a client's dreams. Both of these methods can reveal thoughts or anxieties that remain in the unconscious mind, so they can be brought into conscious awareness (Sue et al., 2017).

Over time, Freud's original theory and thus the psychodynamic perspective have expanded to include newer models, including object relations theory and self-psychology. Contemporary psychodynamic approaches are also informed by attachment theory (Delgado et al., 2015). For example, psychodynamic models rooted in attachment theory are based on the belief that experiences with caregivers during early childhood can influence adult relationships and lead to interpersonal conflict (Sue et al., 2017). Object relations theory offers a similar perspective, positing that caregivers in early childhood serve as "objects," and relationships with these caregivers affect how a child comes to see themselves and others internally. Children develop object relations based on their early experiences with caregivers, forming internal emotional and cognitive models that influence how they relate to themselves and others. These patterns of object relations continue into adulthood (Summers, 2024). Finally, self psychology, based on the work of Heinz Kohut, emphasizes the role of external validation and idealization in the development of a healthy sense of self. This branch of psychology also places a great deal of importance on empathy, viewing it as essential for psychological health (Flanagan, 2021).

CONCEPTUALIZATIONS OF EATING DISORDERS IN THE PSYCHODYNAMIC PERSPECTIVE

It's essential to understand the foundational theoretical concepts that inform the psychodynamic perspective before applying these concepts to eating disorder treatment. Now, having an understanding of the theoretical roots of this perspective, the next step is to learn how this approach conceptualizes eating disorders. The conceptualization varies upon the specific eating disorder in question, as described in the sections that follow.

Psychodynamic Conceptualizations of Anorexia Nervosa

The psychodynamic perspective views anorexia nervosa as arising from a fragile sense of self and an insecure attachment style, in line with modern approaches based on self-psychology and attachment theory (Trombetta et al, 2024). More specifically, psychodynamic theorists conceptualize anorexia as a deficit in the self, which involves difficulty separating one's own needs from others. Furthermore, individuals with anorexia may struggle to integrate their bodies into their sense of self, instead viewing the body as an object separate from the self. The deficits described here are believed to be rooted in attachment insecurity, as well as sociocultural pressures, such as the thin ideal (Amianto et al., 2016).

In addition to considering the role of the self and early life attachments, the psychodynamic modality views symptoms of eating disorders as manifestations of repressed emotional pain. In the case of anorexia, food restriction and extreme fear of weight gain can be a means of avoiding internal conflict that remains in the subconscious (Zerbe, 2015). Finally, it can be helpful to consider anorexia in light of Ronald Fairbairn's endopsychic personality structure, based on object relations theory. Fairbairn's model posits that the ego is relationship-seeking, and in individuals with eating disorders, the experience of emotional deprivation in early life causes the psyche to split into different parts as a coping mechanism. In anorexia nervosa, food represents a rejecting caretaker, which the patient internalizes and then subconsciously punishes themselves via food refusal. In this conceptualization, a patient living with anorexia represses their needs and instead aligns with a harsh, critical internal voice that depicts hunger as shameful (Mohajer et al., 2024).

Psychodynamic Conceptualizations of Bulimia Nervosa and Binge-Eating Disorder

Both bulimia nervosa and binge-eating disorder are linked to impulsiveness and difficulties with emotion regulation. Psychodynamic theorists postulate that in individuals with these disorders, problems in early childhood relationships can lead people to seek comfort from food, thus leading to eating disorder symptoms (Latzer & Stein, 2019).

According to Fairbairn's model described above, trauma and other negative experiences with caretakers in early childhood can create emotional hunger via deprivation. In individuals with bulimia nervosa, the binge-purge cycle represents internal chaos and the inability to consistently self-soothe. Alternatively, in those with binge-eating disorder, food becomes a way to achieve soothing and stability that were absent during childhood (Mohajer et al., 2024).

Psychodynamic Conceptualizations of Other Eating Disorders

While there is existing literature related to psychodynamic conceptualizations of anorexia nervosa, bulimia nervosa, and binge-eating disorder, there is less scholarly work on the conceptualization of other eating disorders via this orientation. For example, avoidant/restrictive food intake disorder (ARFID), is a relatively new diagnosis (American Psychiatric Association, 2016), with less literature related to its theoretical conceptualizations. However, ARFID can be conceptualized according to general principles in the psychodynamic perspective. Based on psychodynamic theory, it can be seen as a manifestation of early developmental problems in the caregiver-child relationship. These problems can lead to difficulties with emotion regulation, as well as sensitivity to internal and external stimuli, resulting in restrictive eating patterns as a way to manage the distress associated with eating (Moberg et al., 2021).

PSYCHODYNAMIC TREATMENT STRATEGIES FOR EATING DISORDERS

Based on the existing literature, it is appropriate to conceptualize eating disorders according to psychodynamic perspectives; given this fact, psychodynamic interventions can also be employed in eating disorder treatment. Psychodynamic therapy modalities, when applied to eating disorders, explore unconscious conflicts, early developmental experiences, and relational patterns that maintain eating disorder symptoms. The ultimate goal in this modality is to help patients gain insight into the underlying dynamics and emotional processes that contribute to the eating disorder. Some clinicians treating eating disorders may utilize a specific psychodynamic modality called focal psychodynamic therapy. This is a manualized approach consisting of 40-50 sessions and emphasizing interpersonal relationships and the achievement of insight (Trombetta et al., 2024).

Beyond the overarching goals of psychodynamic therapy for eating disorders, there are some specific features of this modality that can move patients toward healing. For example, psychodynamic therapy begins with the development of a strong therapeutic alliance, which is the working relationship between patient and therapist. The development of the therapeutic alliance occurs via empathetic listening and the display of respect for the patient. These factors increase the patient's comfort with sharing concerns, thoughts, and emotions with the therapist. After the working alliance is formed, the clinician and patient collaborate to determine the nature of internal conflicts contributing to eating disorder symptoms (Murphy et al., 2005). Another important component of the therapeutic relationship is the occurrence of transference and countertransference during therapy sessions. Transference occurs when the therapist calls attention to ways the patient, during sessions, repeats with the therapist what the patient has experienced in previous relationships (Zerbe, 2015). For example, a patient with unresolved trauma related to her father's absence may view a male therapist as being distant and aloof, when these feelings actually relate to what she feels about her father. On the other hand, countertransference refers to the therapist's reactions to the patient, which may reflect areas that require further exploration (Zerbe, 2015).

Another central concept in psychodynamic therapy is the examination of defense mechanisms, which, as discussed earlier in this chapter, are unconscious strategies employed to manage internal conflicts and emotional distress (Sue et al., 2017). In the context of eating disorders, behaviors such as restrictive eating, bingeing, and purging can be understood as unhealthy defense mechanisms against overwhelming emotions or unmet needs. For instance, restrictive eating may serve as a means to exert control in the face of perceived chaos; while binging and purging might help a patient to regulate intense feelings of shame or guilt. By bringing these unconscious processes to awareness, therapy aims to replace these defenses with healthier coping mechanisms (Friederich et al., 2023).

Furthermore, psychodynamic therapy explores the role of early attachment experiences in the development of eating disorders. Insecure or disrupted attachments can lead to difficulties in emotion regulation and self-concept, which may manifest as disordered eating behaviors. By revisiting and working through these early relational experiences, therapy aims to heal attachment wounds and promote healthier ways of relating to oneself and others (Friederich et al., 2023).

In summary, psychodynamic psychotherapy addresses eating disorders by uncovering and resolving the unconscious conflicts and relational patterns that underlie maladaptive behaviors. Through techniques such as exploring defense mechanisms, analyzing transference and countertransference, and fostering a strong therapeutic alliance, this approach seeks to facilitate lasting change and psychological growth.

CASE STUDIES USING THE PSYCHODYNAMIC PERSPECTIVE

To solidify understanding of how the psychodynamic perspective applies to eating disorder treatment, it's helpful to examine case studies in which a patient is exposed to this modality. Applications of the psychodynamic modality in the treatment of both anorexia nervosa and binge-eating disorder are described below.

Case Study of Psychodynamic Therapy for Anorexia Nervosa

Delaney, a 19-year-old young woman, was admitted to an inpatient mental health facility with a weight of 64 pounds, approximately 54 pounds underweight. Upon admission, Delaney was severely malnourished, and she showed signs of damage to her liver, kidney, and pancreas. Delaney was in denial of the severity of her low body weight and continued to show extreme fear of weight gain, despite her critical condition. She was diagnosed with anorexia nervosa, and her treating therapist used the psychodynamic modality as follows:

- After building a relationship with Delaney and reviewing her history, Delaney's therapist determined that Delaney's food refusal allowed Delaney to obtain a sense of control in response to early childhood neglect. Her behavior served as a way to punish herself, while also representing a cry for attention. Ultimately, it became clear to the therapist that Delaney's early life experiences led to unresolved relational trauma and a fragile sense of self.
- Guided by the psychodynamic perspective, Delaney's therapist helped Delaney to explore her early childhood attachment experiences, as well as internalized critical voices. This helped Delaney to gain insight into the meaning of her disordered eating behaviors and eventually allowed her to learn healthier ways of coping.
- After 59 days of being hospitalized, Delaney was discharged at a healthier weight of 105 pounds. She agreed to return to the hospital if her weight dropped below 100 pounds. Because psychodynamic therapy is typically a long-term modality, Delaney continued to see a therapist on an outpatient basis. Over time, she maintained her progress, and her weight stabilized.

Case Presentation of Psychodynamic Therapy for Binge-Eating Disorder

Javier is a 35-year-old man seeking treatment after a lengthy history of binge-eating episodes. He has made several attempts to stop binging, but he is unable to control his eating. After being diagnosed with binge-eating disorder, his therapist recommends the psychodynamic modality for his treatment, which proceeds as described below:

- Javier's therapist works to create a trusting professional relationship with Javier. After building a strong therapeutic relationship, Javier and his therapist discuss Javier's upbringing, and it becomes clear to the therapist that Javier grew up with harsh, emotionally distant parents. The therapist concludes that Javier's binge-eating helps him soothe his unmet emotional needs and cope with underlying feelings of inadequacy.
- Throughout the process of therapy, Javier's therapist helps him to uncover subconscious emotional conflicts and explore the symbolic meaning that food plays in his life. Javier comes to understand how his past relationships are influencing his current eating behaviors. The therapist also interprets Javier's transference reactions to give him additional insight into unresolved emotional conflicts.
- As a result of therapy, Javier is able to implement healthier coping strategies, without turning to binge-eating. He develops an understanding of the underlying emotional triggers for binge episodes and is able to use more adaptive stress management strategies.

CONCLUSION

The psychodynamic modality, with its emphasis on attachment insecurity, sense of self, and unresolved emotional conflicts, can be useful in the treatment of eating disorders. According to psychodynamic theory, disordered eating behavior can serve as an unhealthy coping mechanism for relational issues or unresolved emotional pain. By bringing these issues to light in therapy, patients can gain insight and learn healthier ways of coping with distress and pain (Amianto et al., 2016; Mohajer et al., 2024; Zerbe, 2015).

Clinicians who utilize psychodynamic methods should be aware of the potential limits of this modality in eating disorder treatment. While there is evidence that psychodynamic therapy can be effective for treating those with eating disorders, additional research is necessary. The current evidence base isn't large, and quality studies, primarily randomized controlled trials, are lacking. Future research should determine the specific psychodynamic techniques that are beneficial for symptom improvement (Abbate-Daga et al., 2016). In theory, psychodynamic modalities seem appropriate for treating eating disorders, but clinicians using the psychodynamic modality should carefully evaluate patient progress, adjusting treatment as necessary to ensure that it remains evidence-based for each patient.

REFERENCES

Abbate-Daga, G., Marzola, E., Amianto, F., & Fassino, S. (2016). A comprehensive review of psychodynamic treatments for eating disorders. *Eating and Weight Disorders*, *21*(4), 553–580. DOI: 10.1007/s40519-016-0265-9 PMID: 26980319

American Psychiatric Association. (2016). *Feeding and eating disorders: DSM-5 selections*. American Psychiatric Association.

Amianto, F., Northoff, G., Abbate Daga, G., Fassino, S., & Tasca, G. A. (2016). Is anorexia nervosa a disorder of the self? A psychological approach. *Frontiers in Psychology*, *7*(849). Advance online publication. DOI: 10.3389/fpsyg.2016.00849 PMID: 27378967

Delgado, S. V., Strawn, J. R., & Pedapati, E. (2015). *Contemporary psychodynamic psychotherapy for children and adolescents: Integrating intersubjectivity and neuroscience*. Springer. DOI: 10.1007/978-3-642-40520-4

Farrell, E. (1995). Psychoanalytic understanding. In Young, R. M. (Ed.), *Lost for words: The psychoanalysis of anorexia and bulimia*. Psychoanalysis and Psychotherapy., Retrieved from https://www.psychoanalysis-and-therapy.com/human_nature/farrell/chap2.html

Flanagan, L. M. (2021). The theory of self psychology. In Berzoff, J., Flanagan, L. M., & Hertz, P. (Eds.), *Inside out and outside in: Psychodynamic clinical theory and psychopathology in contemporary multicultural contexts* (5th ed., pp. 125–151). Rowman & Littlefield.

Friederich, H.-C., Zipfel, S., & Wild, B. (2023). Psychodynamic Therapies and Eating Disorders. In *Eating Disorders* (pp. 1–20). Springer., DOI: 10.1007/978-3-030-97416-9_66-1

Gabbard, G. O. (2004). *Long-term psychodynamic psychotherapy: A basic text*. American Psychiatric Publishing.

Latzer, Y., & Stein, D. (2019). Introduction: Novel perspectives on the psychology and psychotherapy of eating disorders. *Journal of Clinical Psychology*, *75*(8), 1369–1379. DOI: 10.1002/jclp.22786 PMID: 30995356

Moberg, L. T., Solvang, B., Sæle, R. G., & Myrvang, A. D. (2021). Effects of cognitive-behavioral and psychodynamic-interpersonal treatments for eating disorders: A meta-analytic inquiry into the role of patient characteristics and change in eating disorder-specific and general psychopathology in remission. *Journal of Eating Disorders*, *9*(74), 74. Advance online publication. DOI: 10.1186/s40337-021-00430-8 PMID: 34174942

Mohajer, R., Dick, S., Salinas, N. D., & Zolnikov, T. R. (2024). To eat, or not to eat? A psychoanalytic view on the food–parent. *British Journal of Psychotherapy*, *40*(4), 582–595. https://rave.ohiolink.edu/ejournals/article/4374142. DOI: 10.1111/bjp.12917

Murphy, S., Russell, L., & Waller, G. (2005). Integrated psychodynamic therapy for bulimia nervosa and binge eating disorder: Theory, practice, and preliminary findings. *European Eating Disorders Review*, *13*(6), 383–391. DOI: 10.1002/erv.672

Opland, C., & Torrico, T. J. (2025). Psychodynamic therapy. In *StatPearls*. StatPearls Publishing., https://www.ncbi.nlm.nih.gov/books/NBK606117/

Sue, D., Sue, D. W., Sue, D., & Sue, S. (2017). *Essentials of understanding abnormal behavior* (3rd ed.). Cengage.

Summers, F. (2024). *Object relations theories and psychopathology: A comprehensive text* (2nd ed.). Routledge.

Trombetta, T., Bottaro, D., Paradiso, M. N., Rocchi, M. B. L., Polselli, G. M., & Biondi, M. (2024). Psychodynamic group therapy for eating disorders: A narrative review. *Journal of Contemporary Psychotherapy*, *54*(3), 253–264. DOI: 10.1007/s10879-023-09614-6

Zerbe, K. (2015). Psychodynamic theory of eating disorders. In Smolak, L., & Levine, M. P. (Eds.), *The Wiley handbook of eating disorders*. Wiley-Blackwell., DOI: 10.1002/9781118574089.ch20

KEY TERMS AND DEFINITIONS

Countertransference: In psychodynamic therapy, the emotional reactions of the therapist to the patient

Defense mechanisms: Unconscious methods that patients use to block painful material from conscious awareness

Ego: The layer of personality structure in Freud's psychoanalytic theory that is grounded in reality

Free association: A method used in psychodynamic therapy, in which the patient says whatever comes to mind, to assist with identifying subconscious material

Id: The pleasure-seeking layer of personality structure in Freud's psychoanalytic theory

Psychoanalytic theory: Sigmund Freud's original theory, which viewed internal conflict and subconscious drives as the root of psychological suffering

Superego: The layer of personality structure in Freud's psychoanalytic theory that emphasizes morality

Therapeutic alliance: The strong working relationship between clinician and patient, which is viewed as essential in psychodynamic therapy

Transference: Patient behaviors toward the therapist that reflect the patient's experiences in past relationships

CASE NOTES

Case Presentation of Psychodynamic Therapy for Anorexia Nervosa

Questions

1. What symptoms of anorexia nervosa does Delaney show?
2. How does the approach to Delaney's treatment align with the psychodynamic model?
3. How might Delaney's food restriction serve as a defense mechanism?
4. How, specifically, would Delaney's presentation be explained via the self psychology framework?
5. What factors are essential to Delany's treatment?

Epilogue and Lessons Learned

Delaney shows several symptoms of anorexia nervosa, including low body weight, denial of her condition, and extreme fear of weight gain. The approach employed to treat Delaney aligns with the psychodynamic perspective, because of the exploration of childhood attachment issues, experiences of neglect, and internal emotional conflict. Delaney's food restriction could serve as a defense mechanism, by helping her to block out the pain of early childhood neglect. The self psychology framework would state that Delaney did not receive adequate validation during childhood and thus does not have an integrated sense of self. The factors essential to Delaney's treatment include a strong relationship with her therapist, exploration of childhood experiences and internal conflict, and the gaining of insight into her problems. It was also essential for Delaney to learn healthier coping skills.

Case Presentation of Psychodynamic Therapy for Binge-Eating Disorder

Questions

1. What is the name for the trusting professional relationship the therapist builds with Javier?
2. How does Javier's treatment align with the psychodynamic perspective?
3. How would a psychodynamic therapist describe Javier's object relations?
4. How would Javier's object relations lead him to feel about himself?
5. If Javier displayed evidence of transference in a session with his therapist, how might this look?

Epilogue and Lessons Learned

In the given case example, the trusting professional relationship the therapist builds with Javier is called the therapeutic alliance. Javier's treatment aligns with the psychodynamic perspective, because of the exploration of unresolved emotional conflicts from childhood, as well as the influence of past relationships. A psychodynamic therapist would state that Javier's object relations, and more specifically his representation of his parents, would lead him to internalize others as being harsh and rejecting. These object relations are likely to lead Javier to feel inadequate. If Javier demonstrates transference during a therapy session, he may perceive his therapist as being overly harsh and critical, when these are actually feelings he has about his parents.

List of Additional Sources (for all case presentations in this chapter)

1. Herzog, W., Wild, B., Giel, K. E., Junne, F., Friederich, H.-C., Resmark, G., & ANTOP Study Group. (2022). Focal psychodynamic therapy, cognitive behaviour therapy, and optimised treatment as usual in female outpatients with anorexia nervosa (ANTOP study): 5-year follow-up of a randomised controlled trial in Germany. *The Lancet Psychiatry, 9*(4), 280–290. https://doi.org/10.1016/S2215-0366(22)00028-1

2. Tasca, G. A., & Balfour, L. (2019). Psychodynamic treatment of eating disorders: An attachment-informed approach. In D. Kealy & J. S. Ogrodniczuk (Eds.), *Contemporary psychodynamic psychotherapy: Evolving clinical practice* (pp. 207–221). Elsevier Academic Press. https://doi.org/10.1016/B978-0-12-813373-6.00014-3
3. Winston, T. (2012). Psychodynamic approaches to eating disorders. In J. R. E. Fox & K. P. Goss (Eds.), *Eating and its disorders* (Chap. 17). Wiley-Blackwell. https://doi.org/10.1002/9781118328910.ch17

Chapter 8
Other Individual Approaches to Eating Disorder Treatment

ABSTRACT

This chapter describes other approaches used in individual therapy with patients diagnosed with eating disorders, including behavioral therapy, interpersonal psychotherapy, and person-centered approaches. The behavioral therapy approaches discussed in this chapter focus on modifying external behaviors rather than altering thought patterns. In its discussion of behavioral approaches, the chapter introduces key behavioral modalities including Acceptance and Commitment Therapy, exposure and response prevention, mindfulness-based interventions, and behavioral weight loss programs. Through detailed case examples, the chapter depicts how these approaches promote psychological flexibility, reduce avoidance, and help people to tolerate uncomfortable emotions, thereby leading to a change in disordered behaviors. The chapter also includes a discussion of interpersonal psychotherapy (IPT), a time-limited, diagnosis-focused treatment initially developed for major depressive disorder. It outlines the theoretical foundations of IPT, emphasizing the role of interpersonal relationships in the onset and maintenance of psychological symptoms. The chapter details the structure of IPT, including its focus on four primary problem areas: grief, role disputes, role transitions, and interpersonal deficits. It also discusses the application of IPT to eating disorder treatment. Finally,

DOI 10.4018/979-8-3373-0664-3.ch008

the chapter concludes with a brief discussion of person-centered therapy and its emphasis on providing patients with unconditional acceptance to help them overcome conditions of worth.

INTRODUCTION

Previous chapters on eating disorder therapy within this text have emphasized one particular treatment modality each, primarily because certain modalities are especially unique and warrant attention on their own. For instance, as a comprehensive, manualized treatment, dialectical behavior therapy warrants discussion in its own chapter. The same could be said for cognitive behavioral therapy, which is often lauded as the gold standard among psychotherapy modalities. While previous chapters have discussed one modality each, the current chapter discusses several other individual approaches that may be utilized in eating disorder treatment. This is not meant to suggest that these approaches are in any way inherently inferior; they are just used less often in eating disorder treatment and may not be considered as the first line of treatment. They are, however, among modalities that may be considered to meet a diverse range of patient needs. To ensure that a comprehensive list of eating disorder treatment modalities is discussed, this chapter will highlight behavioral approaches, interpersonal therapy, and person-centered therapy.

BEHAVIORAL APPROACHES IN EATING DISORDER TREATMENT

To those unfamiliar with the nuances of the different psychotherapy modalities, behavioral therapy may sound the same as cognitive behavioral therapy (CBT), discussed in a previous chapter, but there are differences between the two. While CBT incorporates both cognitive and behavioral approaches, the behavioral therapies focus on changing outward behaviors. Behavioral therapies are rooted in behaviorism, which posits that people learn behavior and can therefore learn new behaviors. The aim of the behavioral approaches is to change behavioral patterns that lead to challenges or exacerbate life problems. For instance, behavioral approaches for depression, such as acceptance and commitment therapy, help people choose new behaviors that align with their values, rather than responding inflexibly to internal thoughts and feelings (Fogelkvist et al. 2020). This chapter describes the behavioral therapies, including acceptance and commitment therapy, exposure therapy, and mindfulness-based approaches. It also details behavioral weight loss interventions, discussed in chapter 4, which are beneficial for binge-eating disorder (Grilo, 2017; Grilo & Juarascio, 2023; Palavras et al., 2021). While some of the approaches used in these therapies may also be incorporated into CBT modalities, the author believes the behavioral therapies warrant a separate chapter, as they do diverge in some respects from standard and enhanced CBT treatments.

Acceptance and Commitment Therapy in Eating Disorder Treatment

Acceptance and commitment therapy (ACT) is considered a "third wave" cognitive-behavioral therapy, and it includes behavioral components. ACT focuses on unhelpful behaviors, primarily emotional avoidance and the attempt to control one's internal experiences. Some specific behaviors that fall under these categories include numbing oneself through substance misuse, distracting oneself, suppressing thoughts, or avoiding certain behaviors. According to principles of ACT, avoiding emotions or attempting to control them is maladaptive. The goal of therapy, then, is to teach a person to become more psychologically flexible, which helps them to accept uncomfortable emotions. ACT teaches mindfulness practices and also supports individuals in choosing new behaviors that are more in agreement with their values. Consider a patient struggling with anorexia nervosa, for instance. They may have uncomfortable thoughts, such as believing their body is too large. In this instance, food restriction is seen as an attempt to control this thought. Through ACT, a person could learn to accept the thought rather than trying to control it, while choosing a behavior other than food restriction in response to the thought (Manlick et al., 2013).

Before delving into case studies in which a therapist uses ACT as the primary treatment modality, it's essential to fully understand the theoretical underpinnings of this model. First, ACT incorporates a concept called experiential avoidance, which occurs when people avoid unpleasant internal material, including uncomfortable thoughts and emotions. To combat the problem of experiential avoidance, ACT teaches people to be more psychologically flexible, which means they can become fully aware of their thoughts and feelings, even when they are uncomfortable, and make choices that align with their values. By becoming psychologically flexible, people can choose new behaviors, rather than behaving in a way that rigidly conforms to their thinking patterns. According to the ACT modality, when people view their thoughts as being absolute truths, they succumb to a process called cognitive fusion, which causes them to act in accordance with their thoughts. By learning cognitive defusion, people can learn to accept their thoughts without judgment, and instead choose new behaviors that do not conform to rigid or unhelpful thinking patterns. Where ACT differs from CBT is that the therapist does not attempt to help a person change maladaptive thinking patterns; instead, people learn to accept thoughts through mindful awareness, rather than attempting to control unpleasant thoughts and emotions via rigid behaviors (Fogelkvist et al. 2020).

Case Studies

Having reviewed the general explanation of ACT above, the next step in understanding the use of ACT in eating disorder treatment is to analyze case studies that exemplify how this modality can be used in specific case presentations. Two case studies of ACT in eating disorder treatment follow.

Case Presentation of ACT for Anorexia Nervosa

Emily is 19 years of age, and she has lost a significant amount of weight over the last year, placing her BMI at 17. She has an intense fear of weight gain, and she follows a very restrictive diet, in addition to exercising excessively, to maintain a low body weight. Upon assessment, Emily is found to meet DSM-5-TR diagnostic criteria for anorexia nervosa. After reviewing her case with a supervisor, the clinical social worker overseeing Emily's therapeutic treatment determines that ACT is a suitable fit for Emily. The social worker uses the following interventions, based on ACT principles, in her work with Emily:

- **Development of insight:** Emily has used perfectionistic tendencies, excessive exercise, and food restriction, which the social worker identifies is an attempt for Emily to regulate her anxiety. The social worker helps Emily come to the realization that these strategies may provide short-term relief of anxiety, but over the long-term, they have created eating disorder symptoms, and in consequence, heightened anxiety.
- **Identifying uncomfortable thoughts:** In alignment with principles of ACT, social worker helps Emily to identify her uncomfortable thoughts, which include the belief that Emily must be thin to be valuable. The social worker helps Emily to observe her thoughts, rather than allowing herself to be defined by such thoughts. This helps Emily to develop a more flexible self-concept.
- **Living true to values:** Emily works with her social worker to identify areas of life she valued before eating disorder symptoms took hold, including friendships, academic success, and creative pursuits, including painting and singing. By focusing her attention on returning to these valued areas of life, Emily can engage in new behaviors that do not align with her eating disorder, such as putting time into friendships or focusing on her studies, rather than spending hours per day exercising and counting calories.
- **Mindfulness-Based Skills:** Mindfulness-based interventions included in the ACT modality can help Emily identify her own hunger cues and process her emotions without judgment. Ultimately, mindfulness-based exercises help Emily to regulate her emotions and eat in a way that meets her body's needs.

As noted above, ACT can help Emily to change her behaviors by allowing her to focus on her values, use mindfulness-based strategies, and identify how food restriction and fixation on body image are a response to anxiety and uncomfortable thoughts. The ACT modality, with its focus on modifying psychological inflexibility (Manlick et al., 2013), can be especially beneficial for treating anorexia nervosa, which some experts have described as being rooted in psychological inflexibility (Merwin et al., 2011).

Case Presentation of ACT for Binge-Eating Disorder

Marissa is a 34-year-old woman who reports binge-eating at least three to four times weekly. After episodes of binging, she is highly self-critical and isolates from others. Marissa is embarrassed about how much she eats, and she has gained 50 pounds over the last year due to her binging. She has started to avoid social gatherings involving food, because she cannot control her eating habits and is ashamed of how bad things have become for her. Marissa meets diagnostic criteria in the DSM-5-TR for binge-eating disorder. Marissa sees a clinical psychologist for treatment of eating disorder symptoms, and her psychologist employs the following treatment plan, consistent with the ACT modality:

- **Identifying values:** As a practitioner utilizing ACT, Marissa's psychologist believes that it's essential to identify the things that Marissa values the most. After discussion with Marissa, the psychologist identifies that Marissa most values health, self-care, and connection with others. These values can guide goals related to behavioral change.
- **Cognitive Defusion:** In ACT, the principle of cognitive defusion refers to the act of helping clients simply observe their thoughts without passing judgment on them, so these thoughts have less control over behavior. The goal is not to change unhelpful or negative thinking patterns but rather to minimize the impact of these patterns on behavior, so that a person can choose more adaptive behaviors (Assaz et al., 2018). Marissa's psychologist helps Marissa to simply sit back and observe her common thought of, "I'm disgusting after I binge." Marissa and her psychologist work together to reduce the emotional grip of this thought, ultimately deciding to view it as just a silly voice.
- **Acceptance:** Acceptance is at the core of ACT interventions. In line with this core principle, Marissa and her psychologist collaborate to help Marissa stop avoiding the shame and discomfort she feels after

a binge. Marissa learns to use mindfulness-based practices to help her notice her feelings without judging them, which ultimately helps her to break her cycle of binging.

- **Taking committed action:** Finally, to be successful in ACT, the patient must make behavioral changes. Over time, small changes, such as having a meal with a friend or cooking a balanced dinner, can help Marissa to normalize her eating patterns, so binge-eating is no longer her norm.

In Marissa's case, ACT principles help her to become more accepting of uncomfortable thoughts, which is helpful for managing her symptoms. The improvements made during ACT treatment allow Marissa to change her behaviors to become healthier, rather than continuing the cycle of binging, followed by shame and isolation.

Exposure Therapy in Eating Disorder Treatment

Exposure therapy, with its emphasis on behavioral modification, also falls under the umbrella of behavioral therapies. This modality is considered one of the first choices for treating anxiety disorders, including phobias and panic disorder. The theory underlying exposure therapy is that when people are exposed to a feared stimulus in a supportive environment, over time, that stimulus will no longer create anxiety or fear. Also underlying exposure therapy is the inhibitory learning theory, which posits that people can learn to develop new, non-threatening associations with feared stimuli through exposure. Exposure therapy can be applied to eating disorders because it can be argued that in some cases, food is a feared stimulus, with weight gain representing a feared outcome from exposure to this stimulus. Alternatively, weight gain itself may be the feared stimulus, with resulting feelings of shame and disgust representing the feared outcome. Through exposure therapy, individuals with eating disorders can learn that eating perhaps does not cause intolerable weight gain or other unbearable consequences (Butler & Heimberg, 2020).

Exposure and Response Prevention

Exposure and response prevention is a specific type of exposure therapy that may be beneficial in eating disorder treatment, especially in cases of bulimia nervosa. For instance, when using this modality, a patient with bulimia nervosa may be exposed to a binge episode, and then prevented from engaging in purging. Theoretically, stopping a person from purging should break the cycle of binging and purging, because purging allows the cycle to continue by alleviating the distress a person feels after a binge (Butler & Heimberg, 2020). If a person cannot relieve their anxiety through purging, they will likely stop binging as well, since the cycle will be broken.

Exposure and response prevention, as described above, is heavily based in behavioral theory. For example, the concept of classical conditioning explains how a neutral thought can become anxiety-provoking when paired with a stimulus that usually causes distress (Law & Boisseau, 2019). Consider a person who lives with anorexia nervosa. The thought of gaining weight can become incredibly anxiety-provoking when paired with the image of being teased, ridiculed, or otherwise rejected because of one's weight or body size. In an image-obsessed world, it is not unreasonable to conclude that people have been conditioned to associate weight gain with social disapproval. The concept of operant conditioning can also explain the core beliefs underlying exposure and response prevention. Avoiding certain behaviors can be a form of reinforcement, because doing so allows a person to circumvent anxiety as well. Look back at the example of anorexia nervosa. If eating creates feelings of fear and anxiety, restricting food helps to alleviate these emotions; therefore, food restriction serves as a negative reinforcer. Because food restriction removes fear and anxiety, continued restriction is reinforced, thus perpetuating eating disorder symptoms (Law & Boisseau, 2019). Exposure and response prevention can serve to break this cycle of reinforcement.

In treatment settings, principles of behavioral theory, as described above, can be applied to eating disorder treatment using exposure and response prevention. In this modality, people encounter feared situations with the assistance of a therapist. In eating disorder treatment, this might involve eating a certain food or facing one's image in the mirror. As a person is exposed to a feared stimulus, they are prevented from engaging in disordered behaviors in response. For instance, a person who has consumed a feared food is prevented from then purging or over-exercising to compensate for the food consumption. The belief underlying this sort of therapy is that over time, the person will become habituated to the feared stimulus, which will ultimately lead to a decrease in anxiety. Many exposure therapy methods, including exposure and response prevention, utilize a fear hierarchy, which allows patients to be gradually exposed to feared stimuli. For example, an individual with an eating disorder may start at the bottom of a fear hierarchy, by simply viewing a photo of a feared food. Then, they may move up to watching a video of someone else consuming the food, before trying a bite of the food themselves (Storch & Guzick, 2025).

Case Studies

The following case presentations depict how exposure and response prevention can be utilized in clinical settings for the treatment of eating disorders.

Case Presentation of Exposure and Response Prevention for Bulimia Nervosa

Alejandra is a 23-year-old woman who is binge-eating an average of 4-5 days per week. After binging, she forces herself to vomit to compensate for the calories consumed. Alejandra has identified that high-fat foods, including pizza and ice cream, tend to trigger binge-eating for her. When exposed to these foods, Alejandra cannot control the amount of food she consumes, but afterward, she feels guilty and panicked about how much she has eaten, which leads to purging. Alejandra is worried about weight gain from her binges, and she struggles with poor body image, which controls her moods. Alejandra's therapist supports her recovery through an exposure and response prevention modality, described below:

- **Exposure:** Alejandra and her therapist create a hierarchy of feared foods, beginning with foods that cause some level of distress, and progressing to high-fat foods that cause her extreme distress. Over time, Alejandra gradually exposes herself to these during therapy sessions. First, she practices eating granola bars, and eventually moves up the hierarchy, allowing herself to consume pizza.

- **Response Prevention:** With support from her therapist, Alejandra resists purging after eating her feared foods, even if she has consumed more than intended. The therapist teaches Alejandra strategies for managing her distress after eating. These strategies include grounding techniques and mindfulness-based exercises. Over time, Alejandra is able to break the conditioned link between eating feared foods and needing to purge.

As indicated in Alejandra's case presentation, exposure and response prevention can break the cycle of binging and purging in bulimia nervosa by stopping the reinforcement that comes with purging. Since purging is no longer providing negative reinforcement by removing anxiety or guilt after a binge, the binging is likely to stop as well. This process also supports the concept of inhibitory learning, which posits that eating feared foods will not necessarily lead to intolerable emotional consequences if one avoids purging (Butler & Heimberg, 2020; Law & Boisseau, 2019).

Case Presentation of Exposure and Response Prevention for Anorexia Nervosa

Eric, age 17, has a BMI of 16.1 and follows an extremely restrictive diet. He is terrified of weight gain and avoids high-calorie foods. He has several "food rules," which prohibit him from consuming dairy products or high-carbohydrate foods. Eric also has a distorted body image and refuses to look into mirrors or at photographs of himself, because it's too distressing for him to view his body. Eric's parents, concerned for his well-being, take him to a pediatric day therapy program, where his therapist uses exposure therapy as follows:

- **Exposure**: Eric begins the exposure process by visualizing himself eating feared foods or gaining weight. He then progresses to mirror exposure, in which he stands in front of a full-length mirror and describes how his body appears. With continued support from his therapist, Eric eventually moves up his fear hierarchy and consumes bread and cheeses, both of which are feared foods, during a therapy session.

- **Response Prevention**: After exposures occur during therapy sessions, Eric's therapist supports Eric in adhering to response prevention. She discusses strategies Eric can use after sessions to avoid restricting or excessively exercising.

Over time, the steps above show Eric that he can tolerate the anxiety associated with viewing his body or consuming feared foods. Eric also learns that his anxiety decreases with time, even if he doesn't restrict his food intake. He further realizes that eating certain foods or viewing his body in the mirror do not lead to rejection or unmanageable emotions. By eliminating the negative associations that contribute to his eating disorder, and removing the negative reinforcement that comes with food restriction, Eric is able to recover and restore his weight to a typical range.

Mindfulness-Based Approaches in Eating Disorder Treatment

Mindfulness-based interventions have been briefly discussed above, especially in the context of ACT, but these interventions warrant a separate, more detailed discussion. In addition to ACT, multiple therapeutic modalities incorporate components of mindfulness. In ACT, mindfulness is simply one tool, used alongside several others, for bringing psychological relief. In interventions including mindfulness-based stressed reduction, mindfulness-based relapse prevention, and mindfulness-based CBT, mindfulness is the focal point of treatment. These mindfulness-based treatments teach people to become aware of their experiences, so they can become more attuned to the present. They also help people learn to accept their internal experiences, including emotions, without judgment. While historically under-researched for the treatment of eating disorders, mindfulness-based interventions do show promise (Roos et al., 2021).

Techniques utilizing mindfulness can disrupt the processes that maintain disordered eating. For example, they can break the conditioned association between thinness and social praise that typically occurs in people with anorexia. They can also correct operant learning that occurs in eating disorders. For instance, mindfulness may be helpful for stopping the reinforcing cycle of disordered behaviors, such as restricting food to promote positive emotions or alleviate anxiety. By teaching people to become more accepting of emotional distress, mindfulness-based interventions can promote healthier behaviors, thereby reducing disordered behaviors, such as restricting food or acting on the urge to binge in response to anxiety (Roos et al., 2021).

According to a research review conducted by Mercado et al. (2021), existing research shows that mindfulness-based interventions are beneficial for reducing binge-eating as well as restrictive eating practices. In addition, mindfulness practices are effective for reducing symptoms of binge-eating disorder. Authors of the review explained that mindfulness-based interventions can promote mindful eating, which helps people identify their own hunger and fullness cues. Mindfulness interventions can also improve executive functioning, which can enhance self-control and therefore reduce impulsive overeating (Mercado et al., 2021).

When mindfulness-based interventions are used in behavioral health treatment, the therapist providing services typically begins with psychoeducation to orient the patient to the core principles of mindfulness practice, which include non-judgmental awareness and attention to the present. After an orientation period, the therapist guides the patient through mindfulness-based exercises, such as body scanning and meditation, which train a person to attend to the present and take note of their internal experiences (Crane et al., 2017; Mercado et al., 2021; Zhang et al., 2023).

Case Studies

The following case presentations are helpful for developing an understanding of how mindfulness-based interventions are employed in eating disorder treatment. While avoidant/restrictive food intake disorder (ARFID) is not specifically discussed in earlier parts of this chapter, it is included in a case presentation below. There is limited research on evidence-based interventions for ARFID, but principles of mindfulness can be beneficial for this condition, so it is helpful to view a case presentation involving the use of mindfulness-based interventions to treat ARFID.

Case Presentation of Mindfulness-Based Interventions for Binge-Eating Disorder

Tamia is a 35-year-old woman struggling with repeated binge-eating episodes. During these episodes, she feels as if she has no control over the amount of food she consumes, and afterwards, she feels ashamed. Tamia is worried about the effect the binges are having on her physical and mental health, so she sees a social worker, who helps her learn mindfulness-based practices, as detailed below:

- **Psychoeducation:** Tamia's therapist provides her with information about triggers for binge-eating and how mindfulness can disrupt the cycle of binging.
- **Mindfulness Practices:** During sessions with her social worker, Tamia learns to use body scanning, mindful breathing, and meditation to develop present-moment awareness. This helps Tamia recognize what is going on in her body when she's feeling distressed, and also reduces her urges to binge-eat in response to stress.
- **Mindful Eating Exercises:** Once Tamia develops the ability to attune to the present moment, she is better able to recognize her hunger and fullness cues. This allows her to eat when she is truly hungry, and stop before she loses control and falls into a binge.

In Tamia's case, learning mindfulness practices alleviates symptoms of binge-eating disorder by helping identify her body's hunger cues and regulate her responses to stress. Rather than turning to binge-eating to cope with stress, Tamia can pause, recognize what's happening in her body, and refrain from binge-eating as a coping strategy.

Case Presentation of Mindfulness-Based Interventions for Anorexia Nervosa

Agnes is a 21-year-old college student athlete. As a runner, Agnes has felt pressure to maintain a thin, light physique, and she developed symptoms of anorexia nervosa after dieting to lose what she perceived to be an "extra 10 pounds." She found that food restriction was helpful for relieving the anxiety she had related to her fear of gaining weight and running poorly as a result. Agnes and her therapist work together to help Agnes become more aware of her bodily sensations and emotions, as follows:

- **Psychoeducation:** Agnes' therapist teaches her about the principles of mindfulness and how these principles relate to eating behaviors and body awareness.
- **Mindfulness Practices:** During regular sessions, Agnes practices mindfulness meditation with her therapist to help her become more aware of her thoughts and feelings, and better prepared to process them without passing judgment. Ultimately this also helps Agnes to recognize hunger and fullness cues.
- **Mindful Eating Exercises:** By viewing mealtimes in a non-judgmental and present-focused manner, Agnes learns to view eating as a way to nourish her body, rather than becoming fixated on the anxiety she experiences around food.

After working with her therapist for eight sessions, Agnes improved her eating, reduced her anxiety around food, and developed a more positive body image. She also reported feeling more connected to her body's needs.

Case Presentation of Mindfulness-Based Interventions for ARFID

Mark is a 26-year-old man who has been a picky eater for his entire life. His food selectivity has become so intense that he only eats dry cornflakes, canned soup, and a specific brand of yogurt. Due to limiting himself to these three foods, Mark has begun to experience health problems from inadequate nutrition. Mark recognizes that his health is suffering, but he experiences significant distress related to eating, and he is unsure of how to expand his food consumption to include a wider range of nutritious foods. Mark's psychologist determines that the following mindfulness-based protocol is the best option for Mark's treatment:

- **Psychoeducation**: Mark's therapist teaches him about the principles of mindfulness and provides education on ARFID and the factors that tend to maintain symptoms.

- **Mindfulness Training:** After leaning about basic principles of mindfulness, Mark practices breathing techniques to help him become more aware of the present moment. Breathing techniques also help him to calm himself during eating times. Eventually, Mark is able to apply mindfulness principles to eating, to allow him to focus on the sensory experiences associated with food and tolerate these experiences.

Using mindfulness-based interventions, as detailed above, can help a person with ARFID to become more tolerant of sensory experiences associated with food. Over time, this can help the person to introduce more foods into their diet, thereby reducing symptom severity. While there isn't much research specifically evaluating the impact of mindfulness-based interventions in patients with ARFID, research does support that mindfulness can alleviate eating disorders characterized by avoidance and anxiety (Godfrey et al., 2015). Based on this finding, it's reasonable to use mindfulness-based interventions in patients with ARFID, if these interventions are a suitable fit for a specific patient's needs.

Behavioral Weight Loss Interventions in Binge-Eating Disorder Treatment

Behavioral weight loss interventions focus on the implementation of behavioral and lifestyle changes that promote structured eating patterns, moderate calorie reduction, and increases in physical activity (Grilo & Juarascio, 2023). Research has found that these interventions are effective for promoting weight loss among individuals with binge-eating disorder (Forman et al., 2023).

One behavioral weight loss intervention that can be beneficial for treating binge-eating disorder is the LEARN Program for Weight Management. This program involves individual treatment sessions, during which a patient and therapist work through a treatment manual, discuss self-care, and collaborate to determine a patient's behavioral goals. The program teaches gradual behavioral changes, including modest reductions in caloric intake, improved nutrition, and a commitment to 30 minutes of exercise, five days per week. Patients engage in goal-setting, recording of food intake and exercise completion, and problem-solving during their time in the program (Grilo et al. 2020).

Case Presentation of Behavioral Weight Loss Interventions for Binge Eating Disorder

The following case study outlines how the process of a behavioral weight loss intervention unfolds for a patient with binge eating disorder:

Rachel is a 38-year-old woman who reports binge-eating almost daily after work. She is unable to control the amount of food she consumes during these episodes, and she is so ashamed of her eating habits that she only eats in private and has begun to withdrawal from her usual social activities. Rachel has finally decided to seek treatment, as her BMI has increased to 34.2, and she has developed high blood pressure. Rachel is enrolled in a 16-week behavioral weight loss program, based on the model included in the work of Grilo et al., (2020). While participating in the intervention, Rachel works with her therapist to learn about portion control and the binge-restrict cycle that often occurs with binge-eating. She learns how to self-monitor her food intake and mood and engage in goal-setting, with the support of her therapist. She also works through problem-solving strategies to identify binging triggers and remove environmental cues, such as preferred high-calories snacks, that might trigger a binge. This program is beneficial for Rachel, and after 16 weeks, she is able to reduce her binge-eating episodes to one or two per month, and she achieves a modest weight loss of 12 pounds.

Limitations of Behavioral Therapies in Eating Disorder Treatment

There are potential benefits associated with the use of behavioral therapies in eating disorder treatment, but it's also essential to evaluate potential limitations. One such limitation is the lack of rigorous research with some behavioral modalities. For instance, research with acceptance and commitment therapy has shown some positive effects, but additional research is warranted, because existing studies have utilized small sample sizes, with evidence of selection bias (Onnink et al., 2022). Some of the evidence supporting the use of exposure therapy for the treatment of eating disorders has also been weak, so clinicians should use caution and carefully evaluate outcomes when using this modality to treat eating disorders (Russell et al., 2023).

INTERPERSONAL PSYCHOTHERAPY FOR EATING DISORDERS

Interpersonal psychotherapy has roots in the work of Gerald L. Klerman and Myrna M. Weissman. These researchers analyzed the effects of interpersonal psychotherapy when conducting a clinical trial for major depression. Their interpersonal therapy (IPT) modality is based on the belief that a lack of social support contributes to psychopathology, and conditions like depression have a negative effect on social functioning. The ultimate goal of IPT is to improve social functioning, which in turn alleviates psychological symptoms (Markowitz & Weissman, 2012). While originally developed for the treatment of depression, IPT has a place in treating eating disorders, too. Many patients with eating disorders experience problems with social functioning, and these problems can contribute to the maintenance of eating disorder symptoms (Murphy et al., 2012). Given this fact, IPT can be a suitable treatment for individuals with eating disorders. In the sections that follow, the general features of IPT are discussed, and then its specific application for the treatment of eating disorders is reviewed in detail.

Core Assumptions and Features of the IPT Modality

The core underlying assumption of IPT is that psychological problems, which can include those related to eating disorders, are rooted in interpersonal relationships. For those with eating disorders, the IPT modality would argue that social problems, including role transitions, conflict, and social skills deficits, can play a role in the development and maintenance of eating disorder symptoms. A therapist practicing IPT believes that by addressing interpersonal problems, a person will experience an alleviation of psychological symptoms (Markowitz & Weissman, 2012; Murphy et al.,

2012). The aim of treatment in IPT is to improve interpersonal functioning, which refers to a person's pattern of social and cognitive engagement with other people. The modality also emphasizes the development of social skills, which are those qualities that enable a person to interact and communicate with others. Finally, IPT seeks to help people build higher levels of social support, which is the degree of assistance a person has from others with receiving emotional guidance and needed information (Monterubio et al., 2017).

Fortunately, there is a strong evidence base supporting the use of interpersonal therapy. Its interventions, including psychoeducation, assessment of relationships, and improvements made to social functioning, can be expected to be effective for treating mental health symptoms (Bernecker et al., 2017). Interpersonal therapy is a structured treatment, typically lasting 12-16 weeks and occurring in three phases. During the initial phase, the therapist works with the patient to identify the presenting problem and determine the interpersonal factors that contribute to it. It is common for a therapist to complete an interpersonal inventory, which is a review of a patient's relationship patterns, current relationships, and capability to maintain intimacy with others (Markowitz & Weissman, 2004).

After the initial phase of treatment, deeper therapeutic work can be done. Together with the therapist, the patient works to overcome a social problem, which may involve the loss of a loved one, conflict in a relationship, or transitioning to a new role. If the patient has not experienced any of the three aforementioned problems, the focus of treatment is overcoming social skills deficits. Specific strategies during the middle phase of treatment might include working toward resolving a conflict with a significant other, mourning the loss of a loved one, or processing the emotions that come with a major role transition. During IPT, a patient may also learn how to effectively assert themselves in relationships and overcome patterns such as social isolation. Finally, IPT ends with a review of progress and discussion of the fact that ending therapy is a role transition itself (Markowitz & Weissman, 2004).

Relationship Between IPT and Psychodynamic Modalities

IPT has some roots in psychodynamic theory, explained in the previous chapter. While IPT shares some similarities with psychodynamic therapy, such as an emphasis on the influence of early relationships and emotional expression, it differs in its structure and focus. IPT is more structured and time-limited, concentrating on current interpersonal issues rather than exploring unconscious processes. This pragmatic approach allows for targeted interventions aimed at improving interpersonal functioning and, consequently, reducing psychological symptoms (Markowitz & Weissman, 2004).

Rationale for Using IPT in Eating Disorder Treatment

Other approaches in eating disorder treatment, such as cognitive behavioral therapy or the behavioral methods, emphasize controlling symptoms by normalizing eating patterns or correcting thinking errors that maintain eating disorder symptoms. IPT, on the other hand, seeks to address underlying social factors that contribute to symptom maintenance. The application of IPT to individuals with eating disorders is therapeutically appropriate, as interpersonal dysfunction arising from social anxiety or lack of social skills is a risk factor for eating disorders. More specifically, according to the "interpersonal model of eating disorders," struggling with social functioning can cause low self-esteem and negative emotions, which can lead to the use of eating disorder behaviors as a coping mechanism. This model views engagement in disordered eating as a substitute for social engagement. Thus, improving social functioning eliminates the need to use disordered eating behaviors to cope (Monterubio et al., 2017).

Unfortunately, for those experiencing eating disorders and social dysfunction, disordered eating behaviors can worsen social functioning, leading to a vicious cycle in which disordered eating worsens as a person attempts to cope with social isolation and other interpersonal problems. So, dysfunction in the social realm not only increases the risk of developing an eating disorder; it also serves to maintain the eating disorder. In IPT for eating disorders, the therapist directly links eating disorder symptoms to areas of social dysfunction within the patient's life, helping the patient to both improve interpersonal functioning and alleviate eating disorder symptomatology (Monterubio et al., 2017).

Research has supported the use of IPT for the treatment of eating disorders. A recent research review revealed that IPT was comparable to cognitive-behavioral therapy for the treatment of these conditions. The research suggests that IPT is most effective for younger patients and those with a lower BMI (Zhang et al., 2024).

Case Studies Utilizing IPT

IPT can be successfully applied in the treatment of eating disorders. The case studies below exemplify the use of this treatment modality with various eating disorder diagnoses.

Case Study of IPT for Treatment of Anorexia Nervosa

Sophia is a 19-year-old college freshman, referred to therapy after losing 30 pounds within her first semester of college. Sophia has been severely restricting her calorie intake, and she has lost so much weight that she no longer has a menstrual cycle. Sophia is a perfectionist who reports significant anxiety related to school. She has an intense fear of gaining weight, and she is socially isolating herself so that she does not feel pressured to eat in front of others. Sophia's therapist, an expert in IPT, identifies the role transition to college as being Sophia's primary problem. She treats Sophia using the IPT modality, as outlined below:

- **Initial Phase:** Sophia's therapist completes an interpersonal inventory with Sophia and learns that Sophia had a close friend group and strong social support during high school. Since leaving her home town to come to college, Sophia has struggled to make new friends. She feels overwhelmed by her school work and is so worried about her grades that she isn't getting out and meeting new people. Sophia's therapist calls attention to the fact that Sophia's current struggles with role transitioning are a type of interpersonal struggle. Sophia agrees and reports feeling lonely and out of place at college, which drives her to obtain some sort of control. This need for control is accomplished through food restriction.

- **Middle Phase:** Sophia and her therapist work together to help Sophia adjust to her college environment. Sophia discusses her feelings of grief surrounding the loss of her high school friends and identity. With the encouragement of her therapist, Sophia joins a study group on campus to help her connect with like-minded peers. The therapist also role-plays with Sophia during sessions, to give her practice with initiating conversations with peers. Sophia discusses the role that food restriction plays in her life and comes to the realization that controlling her eating helps her to feel more competent. Sophia's therapist is able to gently call Sophia's attention to how her eating behaviors are connected to a lack of social support, which can be better addressed by reaching out to peers and professors.
- **Termination Phase:** As Sophia approaches the end of her time in therapy, she experiences less social isolation and has begun eating in the campus cafeteria with peers. She is able to recognize that her food restriction was a coping mechanism for feeling left out and struggling to form connections with others on campus. Sophia's BMI improves slightly by the end of therapy, and she attends occasional follow-up sessions with her therapist for support after regular weekly sessions end.

Case Study of IPT for Treatment of Bulimia Nervosa

Natasha is a 28-year-old graphic designer who has come to treatment because she is unable to stop from engaging in repeated episodes of binge-eating. During these episodes, she consumes several days' worth of food in one sitting, and afterwards she feels entirely disgusted with herself. To cope with the shame of the binge episode, she forces herself to vomit. When she presents to treatment, Natasha reports feelings of shame around eating as well as strained communication with her live-in partner, Natalia. With social problems identified as contributing to Natasha's cycle of binging and purging, her therapist carries out IPT as follows:

- **Initial Phase:** After completing an interpersonal inventory with Natasha, it becomes clear that her relationship with her partner,

Natalia, is deteriorating. Natasha reports frequent arguments with Natalia, and she feels her emotional needs are not met. Natasha is able to identify that she tends to binge-eat after conflict and when she feels misunderstood. Natasha also resents her partner's long work hours and lack of presence in the home.

- **Middle Phase**: Natasha works with her therapist to explore her own dysfunctional communication patterns, which involve passive-aggressiveness, unmet expectations, and conflict avoidance. In therapy sessions, Natasha learns strategies for expressing herself more directly. This helps Natasha to grow more comfortable with approaching her partner about her emotional needs. Over time, the frequency of binge-purge episodes decreases. Natasha's therapist helps her to see the link between her eating disorder behaviors and instances of her feeling unheard or dismissed by her partner. Natasha is able to learn alternative coping strategies, such as journaling, when these instances occur.
- **Termination phase:** As the end of treatment nears, Natasha has significantly reduced the frequency of binging and purging. Her binge-purge episodes have declined from four episodes per week, on average, to just two episodes per month. Her relationship with Natalia also improves, because Natasha is able to express her needs directly.

Case Study of IPT for Treatment of Binge-Eating Disorder

Juan is a 45-year-old IT consultant, and he seeks the help of an eating disorder therapist after struggling for several years with binge-eating episodes. Juan discloses to his therapist that he often consumes thousands of calories while alone in the evening. In the middle of these episodes, Juan feels as if he cannot stop eating, and he eats to the point of extreme physical discomfort. Afterward, he feels extremely guilty and experiences hatred for his body. Given Juan's loneliness and lack of social engagement, the following IPT protocol is appropriate for his treatment:

- **Initial Phase**: Juan's interpersonal inventory reveals almost no social engagement. Juan is estranged from his family of origin, and he has no close friends. Juan works long hours as an IT consultant and enjoys his work, but he spends little time in leisure or social activities outside of work. Juan's therapist recognizes that Juan has a long history of social withdrawal and difficulty forming relationships.

- **Middle Phase:** The therapist works with Juan to help him identify when his social disconnection began. Juan realizes that he has also been more of a "loner," and food has been a source of comfort for him. Juan's therapist encourages him to carry out some behavioral experiments, such as attending a local fitness class, where Juan can interact with others without much pressure. Juan practices conversational openers during his therapy sessions and also processes social experiences with his therapist. Despite feeling some discomfort with social interaction, Juan slowly learns to connect with others. Binge episodes become less frequent, especially on days when Juan can interact with other people.
- **Termination Phase:** By the end of therapy, Juan feels more confident starting conversations with others, and he isn't binging as often at night. Juan also reconnected with an old friend via social media, and this gave him momentum for developing other friendships, as well. Juan realizes that loneliness, rather than hunger, drives his binges, and he is committed to continuing to socially engage in order to build confidence and avoid binging as a means of comfort.

Limitations of Interpersonal Therapy

Interpersonal therapy shows promise for treating eating disorders, and recent research has established it as comparably effective to cognitive behavioral therapy. However, additional search is needed to clarify the effectiveness of interpersonal therapy for treating individuals experiencing disordered eating. For instance, additional research with larger sample sizes should be conducted to determine how and why interpersonal therapy works for treating eating disorders. Furthermore, because interpersonal therapy is not as widely-used as other methods, such as cognitive behavioral therapy, more work must be done to promote this modality and make it attractive to both therapists and patients as a potential treatment option (Zhang et al., 2024).

PERSON-CENTERED THERAPY IN EATING DISORDER TREATMENT

Person-centered approaches to eating disorder treatment have been criticized as being inadequate for meeting the needs of patients with formal diagnoses (Lakin & Murphy, 2024), but they are worth mentioning here, given the relevance of concepts from the person-centered approach to psychological healing. As the brainchild of the person-centered approach, Carl Rogers, who is grouped among the humanistic theorists, believed that people are driven to achieve their full potential. Rogers did not emphasize psychopathology in his treatment approaches; instead, he worked to help clients grow and thrive without the restrictions imposed by society. Rogers further believed that people experience distress when subjected to conditional positive regard, which occurs when important people, such as friends, parents, or significant others, provide love only when someone meets their standards. Therefore, Rogers argued that people could reach their full potential when exposed to unconditional positive regard, which develops when people feel loved and respected for who they authentically are. In person-centered therapy, growth occurs when therapists provide an environment of acceptance and nonjudgmental understanding, in line with the concept of unconditional positive regard (Sue et al., 2017). At its core, person-centered therapy is also a phenomenological approach, meaning it seeks to understand the world as patients experience it, with the therapist showing empathetic understanding of the patient's internal experience (Yao & Kabir, 2023).

Some emerging research suggests that person-centered approaches are applicable to individuals living with eating disorders. One recent study with patients diagnosed with anorexia found evidence that these patients felt compelled to obtain positive regard from others by behaving in ways that were seen as pleasing. More specifically, these patients reported that maintaining a certain appearance was more likely to bring positive regard from others. Some participants even reported that they equated being "thin" with being a "good girl." Study authors concluded that for those with eating disorders, the desire for positive regard from others can override hunger, leading to eating disorder symptoms (Lakin & Murphy, 2024).

One of the drawbacks to the person-centered approach to eating disorder treatment is that there is limited research on its effectiveness; however, the emphasis on a supportive, accepting therapeutic environment in the person-centered modality has the potential to be beneficial. Research with individuals in eating disorder recovery has shown that they value the relationships they have with clinical treatment providers, especially when they feel that these providers listen to them. This aligns with the concept of the accepting, nonjudgmental therapeutic environment provided by the person-centered therapist. Furthermore, individuals in recovery have reported striving for personal growth during the recovery process, which also aligns well with the person-centered approach (Wetzler et al. 2020).

Given the lack of research on person-centered approaches to eating disorder treatment, there are few specific guidelines for carrying out this modality with individuals in eating disorder recovery. However, the basic principles from Roger's person-centered modality can be extrapolated to eating disorder treatment. For example, an eating disorder therapist operating from a person-centered standpoint should be intentional about creating a supportive therapeutic environment, in which patients feel accepted and understood. Furthermore, the focus of person-centered eating disorder treatment is likely to be on overcoming conditions of worth, such as the belief that one will not be loved unless they conform to ideal body standards, such as being thin, lean, and attractive. That being said, the truth is that regardless of the primary modality a therapist uses in treatment, there should always be a commitment to conveying acceptance toward and nonjudgmental understanding of patients. In this sense, it could be argued that the person-centered approach should underlie and work alongside any therapy modality a clinician uses.

Case Presentation of Person-Centered Therapy for Anorexia Nervosa

As stated above, there are few specific guidelines for applying person-centered approaches to eating disorder treatment, but the following case study illustrates how a therapist might follow this approach for a patient with anorexia nervosa:

Sophie is a 20-year-old college student diagnosed with anorexia nervosa. She restricts her food intake severely and engages in excessive exercise. Sophie describes a constant "inner critic" that tells her she must stay thin to remain worthy of approval from others. She experiences intense shame if she eats "too much" and often feels that her value depends on being the "perfect daughter" and high-achieving student. In her sessions, Sophie's therapist adopts a ***non-directive, phenomenological stance,*** focusing on Sophie's lived experience rather than her diagnostic label. The therapist demonstrates empathy by reflecting Sophia's feelings of shame back to her in a way that makes her feel understood. Furthermore, the therapist accepts Sophia fully, even when she is critical toward herself or hesitant to open up during sessions. As she becomes more comfortable with her therapist, Sophie is able to explore how conditions of worth from family have led her to believe that she is worthy only if she is thin. Sophie eventually learns to focus on her own needs, rather than on others' expectations.

CONCLUSION

Behavioral interventions, interpersonal psychotherapy, and the person-centered approach can all be useful in eating disorder treatment. Some of the behavioral techniques discussed here may also be incorporated in CBT modalities, but the behavioral interventions can also be used as standalone treatments, so they warrant separate discussion. Third-wave behavioral therapies such as Acceptance and Commitment Therapy can increase psychological flexibility and help people to shift away from rigid, disordered behaviors, and instead choose new actions that align with their values (Fogelkvist et al., 2020; Manlick et al., 2013). Similarly, exposure-based strategies, including exposure and response prevention, can interrupt the fear and reinforcement patterns that maintain disordered eating, which can reduce anxiety and help people to face feared stimuli, such as foods, body-viewing, or weight gain (Butler & Heimberg, 2020; Law & Boisseau, 2019). Mindfulness-based approaches complement these treatments by encouraging present-moment awareness and nonjudgmental acceptance of internal experiences, which can be especially beneficial for those struggling with binge-eating or restrictive eating patterns (Roos et al., 2021; Mercado et al., 2021). Finally, behavioral weight loss interventions provide structure for individuals with binge-eating disorder, helping them to make lifestyle changes that reduce binging and promote physical activity (Forman et al., 2023; Grilo et al., 2020). There are a variety of behavioral interventions that can be implemented in eating disorder treatment, and the best intervention depends on a patient's unique needs.

Furthermore, interpersonal therapy is a suitable treatment modality for some individuals with eating disorders, because of the link between interpersonal dysfunction and eating disorder symptoms. Patients who present to treatment with interpersonal problems, such as social isolation, relationship conflict, the loss of a loved one, or a major life transition, may benefit from the IPT modality. By improving the quality of their relationships and social functioning, individuals with eating disorders can enjoy healthy, fulfilling social connections, rather than turning to binging or food restriction as a way to cope with interpersonal problems (Monterubio et al., 2017; Murphy et al., 2012).

Person-centered approaches may also have a place in eating disorder treatment, but they are less-researched than other modalities (Lakin & Murphy, 2024). Nonetheless, like the other modalities discussed in this chapter, the person-centered approach has potential benefits, in spite of its weaknesses. Some patients may benefit from a purely person centered approach, whereas most are likely to experience positive effects when working with a therapist who displays the traits of empathy and unconditional acceptance that are inherent in the person-centered perspective.

REFERENCES

Assaz, D. A., Roche, B., Kanter, J. W., & Oshiro, C. K. B. (2018). Cognitive defusion in Acceptance and Commitment Therapy: What are the basic processes of change? *The Psychological Record*, *68*, 405–418. https://doi.org/10.1007/s40732-017-0254-z

Bernecker, S. L., Coyne, A. E., Constantino, M. J., & Ravitz, P. (2017). For whom does interpersonal psychotherapy work? A systematic review. *Clinical Psychology Review*, *56*, 82–93. DOI: 10.1016/j.cpr.2017.07.001 PMID: 28710917

Butler, R. M., & Heimberg, R. G. (2020). Exposure therapy for eating disorders: A systematic review. *Clinical Psychology Review*, *78*, 101851. https://doi.org/10.1016/j.cpr.2020.101851

Crane, R. S., Brewer, J., Feldman, C., Kabat-Zinn, J., Santorelli, S., Williams, J. M. G., & Kuyken, W. (2017). What defines mindfulness-based programs? The warp and the weft. *Psychological Medicine*, *47*(6), 990–999. DOI: 10.1017/S0033291716003317

Fogelkvist, M., Gustafsson, S. A., Kjellin, L., & Parling, T. (2020). Acceptance and Commitment Therapy to reduce eating disorder symptoms and body image problems in patients with residual eating disorder symptoms: A randomized controlled trial. *Body Image*, *32*, 155–166. DOI: 10.1016/j.bodyim.2020.01.002

Forman, E. M., Evans, B. C., Berry, M. P., Lampe, E. W., Chwyl, C., & Zhang, F. (2023). Behavioral weight loss outcomes in individuals with binge-eating disorder: A meta-analysis. *Obesity (Silver Spring, Md.)*, *31*(8), 1981–1995. DOI: 10.1002/oby.23790

Godfrey, K. M., Gallo, L. C., & Afari, N. (2015). Mindfulness-based interventions for binge eating: A systematic review and meta-analysis. *Journal of Behavioral Medicine*, *38*(2), 348–362. https://doi.org/10.1007/s10865-014-9610-5

Grilo, C. M. (2017). Psychological and behavioral treatments for binge-eating disorder. *The Journal of Clinical Psychiatry*, *78*(Suppl 1), 20–24.

Grilo, C. M., & Juarascio, A. (2023). Binge-eating disorder interventions: Review, current status, and implications. *Current Obesity Reports*, *12*(3), 406–416. DOI: 10.1007/s13679-023-00517-0

Grilo, C. M., White, M. A., Ivezaj, V., & Gueorguieva, R. (2020). Randomized controlled trial of behavioral weight loss and stepped care for binge-eating disorder: 12-month follow-up. *Obesity (Silver Spring, Md.)*, *28*(11), 2116–2124. https://doi.org/10.1002/oby.22957

Lakin, J., & Murphy, D. (2024). A pilot qualitative study of a person-centered approach to eating in women. *Person-Centered and Experiential Psychotherapies*, *23*(4), 512–530. https://doi.org/10.1080/14779757.2023.2273474

Law, C., & Boisseau, C. L. (2019). Exposure and response prevention in the treatment of obsessive-compulsive disorder: Current perspectives. *Psychology Research and Behavior Management*, *12*, 1167–1174. DOI: 10.2147/PRBM.S211117

Manlick, C. F., Cochran, S. V., & Koon, J. (2013). Acceptance and commitment therapy for eating disorders: Rationale and literature review. *Journal of Contemporary Psychotherapy*, *43*(2), 115–122. https://doi.org/10.1007/s10879-012-9223-7

Markowitz, J. C., & Weissman, M. M. (2004). Interpersonal psychotherapy: Principles and applications. *World Psychiatry; Official Journal of the World Psychiatric Association (WPA)*, *3*(3), 136–139. https://www.ncbi.nlm.nih.gov/pmc/articles/PMC1414693/ PMID: 16633477

Markowitz, J. C., & Weissman, M. M. (2012). Interpersonal psychotherapy: Past, present and future. *Clinical Psychology & Psychotherapy*, *19*(2), 99–105. DOI: 10.1002/cpp.1774 PMID: 22331561

Mercado, D., Robinson, L., Gordon, G., Werthmann, J., Campbell, I. C., & Schmidt, U. (2021). The outcomes of mindfulness-based interventions for obesity and binge eating disorder: A meta-analysis of randomised controlled trials. *Appetite*, *166*, 105464. DOI: 10.1016/j.appet.2021.105464

Merwin, R. M., Timko, C. A., Moskovich, A. A., Ingle, K. K., Bulik, C. M., & Zucker, N. L. (2011). Psychological inflexibility and symptom expression in anorexia nervosa. *Eating Disorders*, *19*(1), 62–82. https://doi.org/10.1080/10640266.2011.533606

Monterubio, G. E., Fitzsimmons-Craft, E. E., & Wilfley, D. E. (2017). Interpersonal dysfunction as a risk factor for eating disorders. In Wade, T. (Ed.), *Encyclopedia of feeding and eating disorders* (pp. 1–4). Springer., DOI: 10.1007/978-981-287-104-6_29

Murphy, R., Straebler, S., Basden, S., Cooper, Z., & Fairburn, C. G. (2012). Interpersonal psychotherapy for eating disorders. *Clinical Psychology & Psychotherapy*, *19*(2), 150–158. DOI: 10.1002/cpp.1780 PMID: 22362599

Onnink, C. M., Konstantinidou, Y., Moskovich, A. A., Karekla, M. K., & Merwin, R. M. (2022). Acceptance and commitment therapy (ACT) for eating disorders: A systematic review of intervention studies and call to action. *Journal of Contextual Behavioral Science*, *26*, 11–28. https://doi.org/10.1016/j.jcbs.2022.08.005

Palavras, M. A., Hay, P., Mannan, H., da Luz, F. Q., Sainsbury, A., Touyz, S., & Claudino, A. M. (2021). Integrated weight loss and cognitive behavioural therapy (CBT) for the treatment of recurrent binge eating and high body mass index: A randomized controlled trial. *Eating and Weight Disorders*, *26*(1), 249–262. https://doi.org/10.1007/s40519-020-00950-7

Roos, C. R., Sala, M., Kober, H., Vanzhula, I. A., & Levinson, C. A. (2021). Mindfulness-based interventions for eating disorders: The potential to mobilize multiple associative-learning change mechanisms. *International Journal of Eating Disorders*, *54*(9), 1601–1607. DOI: 10.1002/eat.23564

Russell, H., Aouad, P., Le, A., Marks, P., & Maloney, D.National Eating Disorder Research Consortium, Touyz, S., & Maguire, S. (2023). Psychotherapies for eating disorders: Findings from a rapid review. *Journal of Eating Disorders*, *11*(1), 175. Advance online publication. DOI: 10.1186/s40337-023-00886-w

Storch, E. A., & Guzick, A. G. (2025). *Childhood obsessive-compulsive and related disorders: Assessment and treatment*. Routledge.

Sue, D., Sue, D. W., Sue, D., & Sue, S. (2017). *Essentials of understanding abnormal behavior* (3rd ed.). Cengage.

Wetzler, S., Hackmann, C., Peryer, G., Clayman, K., Friedman, D., Saffran, K., Silver, J., Swarbrick, M., Magill, E., & Magill, E. (2020). A framework to conceptualize personal recovery from eating disorders: A systematic review and qualitative meta-synthesis of perspectives from individuals with lived experience. *International Journal of Eating Disorders*, *53*(8), 1188–1203. https://doi.org/10.1002/eat.23260

Yao, L., & Kabir, R. (2023). Person-centered therapy (Rogerian therapy). In *StatPearls*. StatPearls Publishing., https://www.ncbi.nlm.nih.gov/books/NBK589708/

Zhang, Z. J., Lo, H. H. M., Ng, S. M., Mak, W. W. S., Wong, S. Y. S., Hung, K. S. Y., Lo, C. S. L., Wong, J. O. Y., Lui, S. S. Y., Lin, E., Siu, C. M. W., Yan, E. W. C., Chan, S. H. W., Yip, A., Poon, M. F., Wong, G. O. C., Mak, J. W. H., Tam, H. S. W., Tse, I. H. H., & Leung, B. F. H. (2023). The effects of a mindfulness-based family psychoeducation intervention for the caregivers of young adults with first-episode psychosis: A randomized controlled trial. *International Journal of Environmental Research and Public Health*, *20*(2), 1018. https://doi.org/10.3390/ijerph20021018

Zhang, K., Xie, Q., Fan, C., Hu, X., Lei, J., Kong, J., Liang, M., Luo, J., & Li, X. (2024). The effectiveness of interpersonal psychotherapy versus cognitive behavioural therapy for eating disorders: A systematic review and meta-analysis. *Clinical Psychology & Psychotherapy*, *31*(1), e2953. DOI: 10.1002/cpp.2953

KEY TERMS AND DEFINITIONS

Acceptance and Commitment Therapy (ACT): A therapeutic modality that uses acceptance and mindfulness-based practices to help people become more psychologically flexible and tolerant of uncomfortable thoughts and emotions, so they can choose behaviors that align with their values, rather than rigid behaviors directed by unpleasant internal material.

Behavioral Weight Loss Interventions: Structured behavioral change programs that help individuals with binge-eating disorder to increase their exercise and normalize eating habits with the support of a therapist.

Classical Conditioning: A learning process in which a previously neutral stimulus becomes associated with a meaningful stimulus, eventually eliciting a similar response as the meaningful stimulus.

Cognitive Defusion: A principle in ACT that refers to a client's ability to separate from their thoughts, so these thoughts do not control their behavior.

Conditional Positive Regard: The experience of being valuable to others only when one meets specific standards.

Exposure and Response Prevention: A therapeutic modality that requires people to gradually confront feared stimuli, with the support of a trained clinician, while avoiding their usual maladaptive responses to these stimuli.

Fear Hierarchy: A list of feared items that begins with items that create a lower fear response, and then progresses to items that create a higher fear response, used in the context of exposure and response prevention.

Interpersonal functioning: How a person engages with others, both socially and cognitively.

Interpersonal inventory: A review of a person's current relationships and relationship patterns, completed in the initial stages of interpersonal therapy.

Interpersonal model of eating disorders: The theory that social problems can cause low self-esteem and negative emotions, which can drive a person to use disordered eating to cope.

Interpersonal psychotherapy: A modality that views interpersonal dysfunction as the cause of psychological problems.

Mindfulness-Based Interventions: A group of therapeutic techniques that emphasize present-moment awareness and non-judgmental acceptance of emotions, thoughts, and bodily sensations.

Person-Centered Therapy: A therapeutic perspective that believes healing occurs in the context of a supportive therapeutic relationship, in which the therapist communicates empathy and unconditional positive regard.

Reinforcement: Something that encourages a person to repeat a behavior, because it offers either some form of reward or an escape from an aversive stimulus.

Social skills: Those traits that are necessary for engaging and communicating with other people.

Social support: The level of emotional guidance and information a person receives from others.

Unconditional Positive Regard: The experience of receiving acceptance from others without being expected to conform to specific standards.

CASE NOTES

Case Presentation of ACT for Anorexia Nervosa

Questions

1. What symptoms of anorexia nervosa does Emily display?
2. How does Emily show evidence of cognitive fusion before treatment?
3. Why is ACT an appropriate modality for Emily?
4. How does Emily become more psychologically flexible with treatment?
5. Does it appear ACT was successful for Emily?

Epilogue and Lessons Learned

Emily shows evidence of anorexia nervosa, because she has symptoms including low BMI, intense fear of weight gain, following a restrictive diet, and exercising excessively. At the start of treatment, Emily is fused to the belief that she must be thin to be valuable, which causes her to act in accordance with this belief by restricting food to maintain a low body weight. The ACT modality is appropriate for Emily, because she has uncomfortable thoughts that are driving her eating disorder behaviors. Emily becomes more psychologically flexible with treatment, learning to accept her uncomfortable thoughts. Once she is able to accept these thoughts, she can focus on alternative behaviors that align with her values, rather than fixating on weight and food restriction. Treatment is ultimately successful for Emily, because she learns to regulate her emotions without turning to food restriction. This allows her to eat in a way that meets her body's needs, rather than succumbing to eating disorder behaviors. Emily's case demonstrates how disordered eating behaviors can serve the purpose of helping a person cope with anxiety and uncomfortable thoughts, albeit in a maladaptive manner. Using ACT principles, a therapist can help a person to identify and accept uncomfortable emotional states without judgment, and choose alternative behaviors, rather than acting in ways that attempt to control an unpleasant internal experience.

Case Presentation of ACT for Binge-Eating Disorder

Questions

1. What indicators of binge-eating disorder does Marissa show?
2. Why is it important for the therapist to discuss Marissa's values with her?
3. Why is cognitive defusion helpful for Marissa?
4. Why is Marissa a good fit for the ACT modality?
5. How did Marissa become more psychologically flexible with ACT treatment?

Epilogue and Lessons Learned

Marissa shows several indicators of binge-eating disorder. First, she is binging three to four times per week at minimum, which meets the criteria for frequency in the DSM-5-TR. Marissa would fall in the mild (1-3 binges per week) to moderate (4-7 binges per week) category based on her frequency of binging. She shows other symptoms, including being unable to control her eating, feeling ashamed, and isolating from others. Discussing values is a core component of the ACT treatment modality. Discussing Marissa's values, which include self-care and health, can help Marissa to see how her binge-eating behavior does not align with her values. This can pave the way for choosing new, values-based behaviors in the future. Cognitive defusion can help throughout his process, because it allows Marissa to separate from her thoughts, including the thought that she is disgusting. By separating from this thought, it will no longer drive Marissa's behavior. Ultimately, the ACT modality is a good fit for Marissa, as she appears to be driven by her negative thoughts about herself, which likely serves to perpetuate the cycle of binging. ACT treatment helps Marissa to become more psychologically flexible, because she can accept the thought of, "I am disgusting," without acting on it. By seeing it as just a silly voice, it no longer has to dictate her behavior, and she can then choose to eat with friends and normalize her eating patterns.

Case Presentation of Exposure and Response Prevention for Bulimia Nervosa

Questions

1. Why is bulimia nervosa, rather than binge-eating disorder, the appropriate diagnosis for Alejandra?
2. What indicators of bulimia nervosa does Alejandra show?
3. Why does Alejandra's therapist begin by exposing her to granola bars, before having her eat her main trigger food of pizza?
4. How does Alejandra's case show evidence that principles of reinforcement are at play in bulimia nervosa?
5. How might the treatment process be different if Alejandra were diagnosed with binge-eating disorder rather than bulimia nervosa?

Epilogue and Lessons Learned

Based on the given case presentation, Alejandra meets diagnostic criteria for bulimia nervosa and not binge-eating disorder, because she is binging and then forcing herself to vomit to compensate for the excess calories. Inappropriate compensatory behaviors occur in bulimia nervosa but not in binge-eating disorder. In addition to her binging and inappropriate compensatory behaviors, Alejandra shows indicators of bulimia nervosa, including loss of control over food consumption, as well as fixation on her body image. In exposure and response prevention, a person is gradually exposed to feared stimuli. In line with this modality, Alejandra's therapist creates fear hierarchy to gradually expose her to feared foods. Beginning with pizza may have been too anxiety-provoking, but beginning with a less feared food like granola bars prevents Alejandra from becoming overwhelmed with the exposure process. During the treatment process, Alejandra is exposed to food items and then prevented from purging. This ultimately stops the cycle of binging and purging, because the behavior of purging is no longer able to provide negative reinforcement by stopping the guilt and panic Alejandra experiences after a binge. In bulimia nervosa, the act of purging serves as a negative reinforcer by removing the emotional consequences of a binge. As long as the negative reinforcement continues, the binge-purge cycle will continue. If Alejandra were diagnosed with binge-eating disorder rather than bulimia nervosa, the treatment process would look a bit different. Since inappropriate compensatory behaviors do occur in binge-eating disorder, the therapist would likely have to prevent the response of binging after exposure to emotional cues, rather than preventing purging.

Case Presentation of Exposure and Response Prevention for Anorexia Nervosa

Questions

1. What indicators of anorexia nervosa does Eric show?
2. Why is exposure and response prevention appropriate for Eric?
3. Eric's therapist begins by exposing Eric to feared stimuli via visualization and eventually exposes him to eating breads and cheeses. What is this process called?
4. How is exposure and response prevention beneficial for Eric?
5. Does it appear Eric has achieved remission of symptoms?

Epilogue and Lessons Learned

Eric shows several indicators of anorexia nervosa, including low body weight, restrictive eating, fear of weight gain, and distorted body image. Exposure and response prevention is helpful for Eric because he shows fear/anxiety of several stimuli, including his image in the mirror, as well as specific foods. By exposing Eric to these feared stimuli and preventing him from restricting food in response, Eric will learn that viewing himself in the mirror or eating certain foods will not create catastrophic consequences for him. When Eric's therapist begins by exposing him to feared stimuli and then progresses to having him eat feared foods in session, she is creating a fear hierarchy. This allows for gradual exposure to feared items. This process is beneficial for Eric, because it removes the negative reinforcement that food restriction provides. This helps Eric to learn to tolerate his anxiety without turning to eating disorder behaviors.

By restoring his weight and stopping his food restriction, Eric will likely achieve remission of symptoms.

Case Presentation of Mindfulness-Based Interventions for Binge-Eating Disorder

Questions

1. What symptoms of binge-eating disorder does Tamia show?
2. How do mindfulness interventions benefit Tamia?
3. Had mindfulness interventions not been beneficial, what alternative intervention(s) from this chapter might you try?
4. How would ACT be different from the mindfulness-based intervention used with Tamia?
5. Do mindfulness-based interventions appear to have been successful for Tamia?

Epilogue and Lessons Learned

Tamia shows symptoms of binge-eating disorder, including repeat binge episodes, loss of control over eating, and feelings of shame. Mindfulness interventions are helpful for Tamia, because they allow her to accept emotions without judgment, so she can stop binging in response to emotional triggers. These interventions also help her to become more aware of her internal experiences, so she is able to act intentionally, rather than binging in response to cues. If mindfulness-based interventions were not beneficial for Tamia, you might try exposure and response prevention; she could be exposed to triggering foods in the treatment setting and then prevented from binging. You might also consider behavioral weight loss interventions, given that Tamia is concerned about her health. ACT would also be beneficial; this intervention also uses mindfulness techniques, but adds in components of learning about cognitive defusion and choosing behaviors that align with one's values. In an ACT treatment modality, Tamia could learn to act in accordance with her values of promoting health, for instance. While there are alternative treatment modalities available, the mindfulness-based approach does appear to have been successful, since

Tamia learns to identify her hunger and fullness cues and to cope with stress without binge-eating.

Case Presentation of Mindfulness-Based Interventions for Anorexia Nervosa

Questions

1. How can we identify from the case presentation that Agnes meets criteria for anorexia nervosa?
2. Would we need any additional information here to make an anorexia nervosa diagnosis?
3. Why does mindfulness benefit Agnes' symptoms?
4. What alternative treatments in this chapter might have been beneficial for Agnes?
5. Why would behavioral weight loss interventions be inappropriate for Agnes?

Epilogue and Lessons Learned

Agnes meets criteria for anorexia nervosa, based on food restriction and fear of weight gain. While these are indicators of anorexia nervosa, we'd also need to know if her food restriction has led to significantly low body weight. Furthermore, we'd need to know if Agnes has a disturbance in body image, fixation on body weight/shape when evaluating herself, or a denial of the seriousness of her low weight. We can infer these things from the description, but if making a formal diagnosis, we'd likely need more information. Mindfulness benefits the symptoms Agnes is experiencing, because it allows her to become more attuned to her internal experiences. It also allows her to eat without passing judgment on the experience or her related feelings, thereby alleviating restriction. ACT is another treatment that may benefit Agnes. It could help her to use cognitive defusion to separate from her belief that she must be thin and light to be a strong runner. ACT would also allow Agnes to act in line with her values, which appear to be centered on running performance. If Agnes values performance, ultimately, she must fuel her body. While Agnes may benefit from ACT, behavioral weight loss interventions would be problematic for her. In anorexia nervosa, restriction and weight loss are the source of dysfunction, so these behaviors should not be encouraged further.

Case Presentation of Mindfulness-Based Interventions for ARFID

Questions

1. How does Mark show signs of ARFID?
2. Why is mindfulness beneficial in cases of ARFID, such as Mark's?
3. Does Mark seem to benefit from this intervention?
4. How would exposure and response prevention help Mark?
5. Why might a clinician use an ACT intervention with Mark?

Epilogue and Lessons Learned

Mark shows signs of ARFID, due to his overall avoidance of most foods and resulting health problems from inadequate nutrition. There is an overall lack of research with mindfulness-based interventions for treating ARFID, but based on the fact that trying new foods can cause anxiety, and thus food avoidance, for individuals living with ARFID, mindfulness-based interventions can be helpful. These interventions can help people with ARFID to accept food-related anxiety without passing judgment on it, which can facilitate a willingness to try new foods. Mark does seem to benefit from this intervention, as it allows him to calm himself during eating times and tolerate the anxiety that comes from eating. Mark could also benefit from exposure and response prevention; this modality could expose him to new foods during treatment sessions and then prevent him from using avoidance behaviors. Finally, a clinician could employ an ACT intervention with Mark to help him reduce the effects that negative thinking patterns, such as food-related anxiety, have on his behavior. ACT could allow Mark to tolerate negative emotions, and choose values-aligned behaviors, like eating to promote optimal health and functioning.

Case Presentation of Behavioral Weight Loss Interventions for Binge Eating Disorder

Questions

1. What symptoms of binge-eating disorder does Rachel show?
2. Why does Rachel's case presentation not meet criteria for bulimia nervosa?
3. Why is behavioral weight loss appropriate for Rachel?
4. Does Rachel still meet criteria for binge-eating disorder after treatment?
5. What goals might you have for Rachel as her clinician?

Epilogue and Lessons Learned

In the given case presentation, Rachel meets criteria for binge-eating disorder, based on repeated episodes of binge eating, lack of control over eating, and shame related to her eating behaviors. She doesn't meet criteria for bulimia nervosa, as there is no indication she is using inappropriate compensatory behaviors, like laxative issue or fasting, following her binges. Behavioral weight loss is appropriate given Rachels's high BMI and high blood pressure. At the end of treatment, Rachel would no longer meet the frequency criteria for a diagnosis of binge-eating disorder. Diagnosis requires that binge-eating episodes occur at least once a week, on average. After treatment, Rachel's binge-eating episodes have declined to one or two per month, so she would be in partial remission. As a clinician, your goals for Rachel might include taking a 30-minute walk daily after work, eating three portion-controlled meals and one nutritious snack per day, and developing a list of coping strategies that do not involve binge-eating.

List of Additional Sources (for all case presentations of behavioral approaches in this chapter)

The following additional readings are beneficial for behavioral health clinicians, physicians, and case managers working with individuals with eating disorders and applying behavioral treatments:

1. Abramowitz, J.S., Deacon, B.J., & Whiteside, S.P.H. (2019). *Exposure therapy for anxiety: Principles and practice.* The Guilford Press.
2. American Psychiatric Association. (2022). Feeding and eating disorders. *In Diagnostic and statistical manual of mental disorders* (5th ed., text rev.; pp. 371–394). American Psychiatric Publishing.
3. Fairburn, C.G. (2013). *Overcoming binge eating: The proven program to learn why you binge and how you can stop.* The Guilford Press.
4. Luoma, J.B., Hayes, S.C., & Walser, R.D. (2017*). Learning ACT: An Acceptance and Commitment Therapy Skills Training Manual for Therapists.* Context Press.
5. Onnink, C. M., Konstantinidou, Y., Moskovich, A. A., Karekla, M. K., & Merwin, R. M. (2022). Acceptance and Commitment Therapy (ACT) for eating disorders: A systematic review of intervention studies and call to action. *Journal of Contextual Behavioral Science, 26*, 11–28. https://doi.org/10.1016/j.jcbs.2022.08.005
6. Parling, T., Cernvall, M., Ramklint, M., Holmgren, S., & Ghaderi, A. (2016). A randomised trial of Acceptance and Commitment Therapy for Anorexia Nervosa after daycare treatment, including five-year follow-up. *BMC Psychiatry, 16*, Article 272. https://doi.org/10.1186/s12888-016-0975-6
7. Rossy, L. (2016). *The mindfulness-based eating solution: Prevention strategies to end overeating, satisfy your hunger, and savor your life.* New Harbinger Publications.

Case Presentation of Interpersonal Therapy for Anorexia Nervosa

Questions

1. What symptoms of anorexia nervosa does Sophia show?
2. What evidence do you have that a role transition is contributing to Sophia's symptoms?
3. What signs of interpersonal dysfunction does Sophia show?
4. In what ways does Sophia's social functioning improve by the end of therapy?

5. Why would interpersonal therapy be a more appropriate option than psychodynamic modalities, discussed in the previous chapter?

Epilogue and Lessons Learned

Sophia shows symptoms of anorexia nervosa, including food restriction, extreme weight loss, and intense fear of weight gain. We can conclude that a role transition is contributing to Sophia's symptoms, because she had a group of close friends in high school, but she now is isolating from others. Sophia shows signs of interpersonal dysfunction, because she is struggling to make new friends and isn't getting out to meet new people. By the end of therapy, Sophia's social functioning improves, because she has joined a study group on campus, is able to eat with peers, and experiences less social isolation. Given Sophia's experiences, interpersonal therapy seems to be a better fit for her than psychodynamic therapy, because she is experiencing social problems in the present. Psychodynamic therapy would be more concerned with uncovering unresolved emotional conflict, which doesn't seem to be the presenting concern with Sophia.

Case Presentation of Interpersonal Therapy for Bulimia Nervosa

Questions

1. What symptoms of bulimia nervosa does Natasha show?
2. Why does Natasha's cycle of eating disorder symptoms appear to have roots in interpersonal dysfunction?
3. What type of interpersonal problem highlighted in the IPT model seems to most affect Natasha?
4. How are Natasha's eating disorder symptoms related to interpersonal dysfunction?
5. Does it appear that Natasha would still meet criteria for bulimia nervosa at the end of treatment? Why or why not?

Epilogue and Lessons Learned

Natasha shows evidence of bulimia nervosa, because she is repeatedly binging and purging. This cycle seems to be related to interpersonal dysfunction, because Natasha reports experiencing strained communication with her partner. Based on this fact, the interpersonal problem that most affects Natasha is conflict. This is one focus of interpersonal dysfunction in the IPT model. It is clear that there is a link between Natasha's eating disorder symptoms and interpersonal dysfunction, because Natasha binges in response to conflict with her partner, especially when it leaves her feeling unheard. At the end of treatment, Natasha is binge-eating and purging twice per month. This would not meet diagnostic criteria for bulimia nervosa, because she is not binge-eating and purging at least once weekly, as required for diagnosis.

Case Presentation of Interpersonal Therapy for Binge-Eating Disorder

Questions

1. How do we know that Juan meets diagnostic criteria for binge-eating disorder rather than bulimia nervosa?
2. What type of interpersonal problem addressed in the IPT model is the focus of Juan's treatment?
3. What evidence do we have that his eating disorder symptoms are linked to interpersonal dysfunction?
4. How does Juan's therapist help him develop stronger social skills?
5. How does improving social functioning help Juan to overcome eating disorder symptoms?

Epilogue and Lessons Learned

Juan meets diagnostic criteria for binge-eating disorder due to his repeated episodes of binge-eating. He does not meet criteria for bulimia nervosa, because he does not engage in compensatory behaviors like excessive exercise or self-induced vomiting after his binge episodes. The primary interpersonal problem addressed in Juan's case is a deficit in social skills. This is the focus of IPT when another interpersonal issue, like grief, role transition, or conflict is not present. We know Juan's eating disorder symptoms are linked to interpersonal dysfunction, because he binges while alone during the evening and has a long history of social withdrawal and struggling to form relationships. Food is also a source of comfort for him, taking the place of social engagement. Juan's therapist helps him develop stronger social skills by practicing conversation-openers with him and assigning experiments, such as attending a fitness class to engage with others. Improving his social skills helps Juan to feel less alone and begin developing friendships with others. Social engagement therefore takes the place of binging, since Juan no longer needs to binge-eat to fill the void of loneliness.

List of Additional Sources (for all case presentations on interpersonal therapy in this chapter)

1. Belik, O., Schultz, J. M., Fairhurst, S., Stuart, S., Vaz, A., & Rousmaniere, T. (2025). *Deliberate practice in interpersonal psychotherapy*. American Psychological Association. https://doi.org/10.1037/0000426-000
2. Frank, E., & Levenson, J. C. (2010). *Interpersonal psychotherapy*. American Psychological Association.
3. Weissman, M. M., Markowitz, J. C., & Klerman, G. L. (2017). *The guide to interpersonal psychotherapy: Updated and expanded edition*. Oxford University Press.

Case Presentation of Person-Centered Therapy for Anorexia Nervosa

Questions

1. What symptoms of anorexia nervosa does Sophie show?
2. Why is empathy important to Sophie's recovery?
3. How do we see evidence of conditions of worth in Sophie's case presentation?

4. How does Sophie's therapist show unconditional positive regard?
5. Why is the person-centered approach appropriate for Sophie?

Epilogue and Lessons Learned

In the given case presentation, Sophie meets criteria for anorexia nervosa, based on food restriction and her need to remain thin. Empathy is important to Sophie's recovery, because it shows that the therapist understands her experiences with shame and feeling the need to be thin to be loved. We see conditions of worth in this case presentation, because Sophie feels she needs to be thin and be a high-achieving student and perfect daughter to be valued. The therapist shows Sophie the unconditional positive regard required for healing by accepting her, even when she is resistant or critical of herself. In the end, the person-centered approach is beneficial for Sophie, because it helps her to overcome conditions of worth in which she feels she must be thin to be loved, which helps her to focus on her own needs.

List of Additional Sources (for the case presentations of person-centered therapy in this chapter)

1. Duffy, K. E. M., Simmonds-Buckley, M., Haake, R., Delgadillo, J., & Barkham, M. (2023). The efficacy of individual humanistic-experiential therapies for the treatment of depression: A systematic review and meta-analysis of randomized controlled trials. *Psychotherapy Research.* Advance online publication. https://doi.org/10.1080/10503307.2023.2227757
2. Rodgers, B., Tudor, K., & Sutherland, A. (2024). *An integrative review of the person-centred and experiential therapy literature on delivering individual video counselling and psychotherapy. Counselling and Psychotherapy Research, 24*, 16–26. https://doi.org/10.1002/capr.12600

Chapter 9
Family-Based Interventions for Eating Disorders

ABSTRACT

This chapter details several family-based interventions for eating disorders. It begins with the Maudsley Method, also called manualized family-based treatment. It discusses other family-focused interventions for eating disorders, including Bowen's family systems theory and Minuchin's structural family therapy, as well as emotion-focused family therapy and strategic family therapy. The author describes the theoretical foundations and core interventions associated with each treatment modality and also discusses their application to eating disorder treatment.

INTRODUCTION

With the exception of dialectical behavior therapy, which includes skill-based groups as a part of treatment, the therapeutic modalities in previous chapters have centered on individual therapy models. The current chapter discusses family-based eating disorder interventions, which can be an essential component of treatment. In some cases, family therapy may complement other interventions, such as individual psychotherapy. In other instances, family-based therapy may be the primary mode of treatment. For adolescents, family-based interventions, and especially

DOI: 10.4018/979-8-3373-0664-3.ch009

Maudsley Family Therapy, are highly effective, and may form the cornerstone of treatment, particularly for treating anorexia nervosa (Brockmeyer et al., 2018). Given the evidence base supporting family therapy models, it's essential to discuss them in detail. In the sections that follow, various family therapy modalities, as well as their applications to eating disorder treatment, are thoroughly reviewed.

THEORETICAL FOUNDATIONS OF FAMILY-BASED TREATMENT (FBT)

There are numerous family-based therapy modalities, but the term "family-based treatment" refers to a specific modality. Family-based methods of treatment, particularly for children and adolescents, have their roots in the Maudsley Method, developed in the 1970s and 1980s at London's Maudsley Hospital. The Maudsley Method does not label parents as culpable for an adolescent's eating disorder. Instead, it views parents as a necessary resource that contributes to a child's recovery. This method represents a divergence from other family treatment modalities, including Minuchin's structural family therapy. While Munuchin's therapeutic model did inform some of the studies conducted with the Maudsley Method, it differed from this method in key ways. First, the Maudsley Method views the adolescent's development as being the primary concern. Rather than addressing family pathology, Maudsley Family-Based Treatment emphasizes empowering parents to help the child with anorexia achieve weight gain and remission. The ultimate aim is for the patient to return to a typical developmental trajectory, rather than continuing with self-starvation, which impedes typical development. So, this model often encourages parents to stop allowing the child with anorexia to make their own food choices (Loeb & le Grange, 2009).

The Process of the Maudsley Method of Family-Based Treatment

Families participating in the Maudsley method for anorexia nervosa undergo treatment in distinct phases. During the first phase, the parents assume control of the child's eating, acting as inpatient treatment providers. The therapist provides support to parents by guiding them through a family meal in-session. During this session, the parents encourage the child to eat at least one more bite of food than the child intended to eat. After the child achieves a minimally acceptable body weight, the family moves into the second phase of treatment, during which the child returns to making their own choices about food. The third phase of treatment then involves moving toward termination and discussing topics related to adolescent development. This family-based treatment is intended to be carried out over 20 sessions, but shorter durations of treatment may also be effective (Loeb & le Grange, 2009).

The Maudsley Method, which is also referred to as manualized family-based treatment, has a strong empirical evidence base supporting its use. According to a review conducted by Lavender (2020), manualized family-based treatment is associated with remission in 35%-45% of cases of adolescents living with anorexia nervosa. Its success rates are so high, in fact, that it is the first choice for treatment in adolescents with anorexia nervosa. Despite the benefits of this modality, not every clinician provides this treatment exactly according to its manual. So, there are numerous modified versions of manualized family-based treatment. While treatment fidelity is important, there are several factors that have been identified as necessary for success, especially in families who have previously failed to achieve remission with treatment. These factors include the therapist providing families with comprehensive education about anorexia nervosa, ensuring that parents are emotionally prepared for the session during which a meal is served, and empowering parents to make decisions that benefit the adolescent's recovery (Lavender, 2020).

As a family-based intervention, the Maudsley Method utilizes some techniques from family systems therapy and structural family therapy, while also incorporating interventions specific to eating disorders. It is believed that this method is beneficial because it exposes the adolescent to feared foods as well as higher weight ranges, helps to normalize hormonal functioning via weight gain, and restructures the family system so that parents are placed in the authority role. By initially giving parents control of the adolescent's eating, the Maudsley Method creates a family environment in which self-starvation is not tolerated, which is why the restructuring of the family system is so essential (Loeb & le Grange, 2009).

Family-Based Treatment for Bulimia Nervosa

While the Maudsley Method, as described above, is designed to treat anorexia nervosa, this method has also been adapted for treatment of bulimia nervosa. One trial with family-based treatment for bulimia nervosa (FBT-BN) found that it led to abstinence from binging and purging in 39% of patients by the end of treatment, but abstinence rates declined over time. Another study found that the abstinence rate at the end of treatment was 39.4%, and it increased to 49% at a 12-month follow-up point. Like family-based treatment for anorexia nervosa, treatments for bulimia nervosa empower parents to stop their children's binge-eating and purging cycle (Loeb & le Grange, 2009).

OTHER FAMILY INTERVENTIONS IN EATING DISORDER TREATMENT

While family-based treatment (FBT) refers specifically to the Maudsley Method, this is not the only family-focused intervention in eating disorder treatment. Modalities like family systems therapy, structural family therapy, strategic family therapy, and emotion-focused therapy may also be used to treat eating disorders.

Family Systems Therapy

In family systems therapy, the family is seen as an interconnected emotional system, in which individual symptoms are indicative of broader relationship dysfunction within the system. Dr. Murray Bowen is credited as the founding father of family systems therapy. According to Bowen, who departed from the psychoanalytic orientation that prevailed during his time, humans organize themselves into emotional systems. As such, when one member of the family experiences a psychological disturbance, it is believed to be a manifestation of a disturbance within the larger family unit. Unlike the psychoanalysts, who viewed the relationship with the primary caregiver, often the mother, as contributing to psychological distress, Bowen asserted that the entire family system– including the nuclear family, the extended family, and other generations– contributed to dysfunction in a person (Palombi, 2016).

Because families operate as an emotional unit, Bowen also believed that each individual experiences a tension between separateness and togetherness in the context of family life. On the one hand, people have a need to be individually separate from their family members, with their own ways of thinking, feeling, and acting. On the other hand, they must maintain some sense of togetherness with their family, causing people to share thoughts and feelings with family members (Palombi et al., 2016). Perhaps the most defining feature of Bowen's theory is his emphasis on anxiety, which he believed arose in response to too much closeness, or at the opposite end of the spectrum, too much distance in families (Brown & Errington, 2024). Beyond this focus, Bowen's family systems therapy is centered on several key concepts, which are described below.

Differentiation of Self

Bowen described differentiation of self as the ability to remain both connected and independent, in a balanced fashion. He also delineated two facets of differentiation of self: intrapsychic differentiation, which involves being able to separate one's own thoughts and emotions, and interpersonal differentiation of self, which requires being able to maintain one's individuality while remaining emotionally connected to others in a relationship. To be healthy, Bowen asserted, a person must have a high level of differentiation of self, as this allows a person to be close to others without losing their individuality. Closely related to the concept of differentiation of self is fusion, which can describe a person whose thoughts and feelings are merged, or a person who is overly sensitive to others' emotional reactions. People who are fused to others will react impulsively to the requests or needs of another person in the family, without much forethought (Brown & Errington, 2024). On the other hand, people who are well differentiated can separate themselves from others' emotions and set healthy boundaries. There is merit to Bowen's focus on differentiation of self, as numerous studies have demonstrated that this concept is linked to psychological health and relationship quality (Calatrava et al., 2022).

Triangles

Another key argument in Bowen's model is that emotions between two people in a family can become too intense, so dyads tend to pull a third party into their conflict, in a process called triangulation. The third party can either take sides in a conflict or serve as a detour for the anxiety associated with the conflict. While triangulation can reduce the discomfort associated with conflict, it often prevents the dyad from resolving their differences. The process of triangulating is also believed to be closely related to the differentiation of self, with individuals higher in fusion having a greater tendency to form triangles (Brown & Errington, 2024).

Nuclear Family Emotional System

The nuclear family emotional system, per Bowen, is the pattern of emotional functioning that occurs within a family in a given generation. These patterns tend to be passed down from earlier generations, so they continue to replay in the family. When tension arises within this emotional system, Bowen stated that families would use one of four strategies to manage it. The first strategy is distance and conflict between the couple. In this cycle, a couple that is emotionally fused will view conflict as an insult, causing an emotionally intense relationship to occur. Over time, they will engage in a pattern of closeness, followed by conflict, which then creates distance. After the conflict is resolved, the couple returns to a state of extreme emotional closeness, and the cycle repeats itself. Another solution for managing conflict in fused families is, quite simply, distance. When people are overwhelmed with discomfort from emotional tension, they can simply remove themselves emotionally or physically from the conflict. Additionally, fusion may cause a dynamic in which one spouse overfunctions, and the other underfunctions. For instance, the more "responsible" spouse may put forth greater effort into caring for the family and home, feeling as if they are compatible with the underfunctioning spouse who puts forth less effort. Over time, this dynamic tends to morph into one in which the responsible spouse becomes increasingly controlling, and the other spouse simply stops participating in the relationship. Finally, fusion can manifest as a child who develops emotional or behavioral problems, such as anxiety. Rather than directly addressing fusion or other conflicts within the family system, spouses may focus on the child, causing that child to absorb the family anxiety (Brown & Errington, 2024).

The Family Projection Process

In the family projection process, emotional and behavioral problems develop in the child as described above. This process occurs when parents "take a detour" from problems in their relationship and instead focus intensely on the needs of a child, often the most poorly differentiated child in the family. Because fixating on a child can relieve marital tension, the couple is driven to continue their focus on the child. This prevents the child from developing their own patterns of thinking, feeling, and behavior. The family projection process is described as being intergenerational, because parents tend to project their own psychological ills onto children, who then become poorly differentiated, and then pass the problem to the next generation (Brown & Errington, 2024).

Emotional Cut-Off

Per Bowen, individuals who cannot cope with intense fusion are likely to engage in a behavior called emotional cut-off, in which they entirely distance themselves from the family of origin in order to start anew. This process can occur via physical distancing, in which a person does not have physical contact with the family of origin. Alternatively, it can occur via emotional cut-off, in which a person withdraws emotionally from the family (Brown & Errington, 2024).

The Multigenerational Transmission Process

Finally, Bowen posited that differentiation is passed down from one generation to the next, causing family problems to persist across generations. This process of multigenerational transmission occurs primarily via the family projection process described earlier, in which a parent projects their anxieties onto a child. Because of his belief in the multigenerational transmission process, Bowen included information about at least three generations of a family when intervening with a presenting problem (Brown & Errington, 2024).

The Process of Family Systems Therapy

In family systems therapy, the primary role of the therapist is to remain neutral while operating within the context of the family's emotional system. Furthermore, the aim of therapy is for family members to reduce their fusion and move toward greater differentiation of self. During the course of treatment, the family systems therapist first seeks to reduce family anxiety, before providing psychoeducation about the systems perspective, so families can understand their problems more deeply. This process unfolds by first alleviating anxiety by asking family members to consider how the presenting problem is part of their relationship patterns, which involve both present and past family systems. Once anxiety is reduced, adult family members learn to differentiate themselves by focusing on their role in the problem and giving up the need to blame or change others in the family. At the end of treatment, the therapist guides adult family members toward differentiating themselves from their families of origin, which in turn benefits the current family system (Brown & Errington, 2024).

Family Systems Therapy for Eating Disorders

There are few studies that apply Bowen's specific family systems method to eating disorders; however, there is extensive support demonstrating that family-focused therapies are effective for treating these conditions. In fact, much of the research with adolescent populations has demonstrated that family therapy is more effective than individual therapy for treating anorexia nervosa. There is less research on the topic of family therapy for bulimia nervosa, but the existing research suggests family-based interventions may be superior to cognitive-behavioral therapy (CBT) (Jewell et al., 2016). While manualized family-based therapy, or the Maudsley Method, is the most well-researched and well-supported method of family therapy for eating disorders, alternative approaches, including those based on Bowen's theory, may be beneficial. One study using principles from systemic family therapy found that a one-week intensive program showed promise for promoting weight gain in adolescents with anorexia nervosa (Rockwell et al., 2011). Additionally, while therapies based on family systems perspectives have been found to be more costly to implement than manualized family-based treatment, family systems therapy may be more beneficial for patients with obsessive-compulsive symptoms (Agras et al., 2014). So, therapy based on Bowen's model may be the most suitable choice for some families.

There isn't an exact model of Bowen's family systems therapy for eating disorders, but researchers have applied Bowen's model to pediatric obesity. For example, in a family in which a child is obese, triangulation may occur, as the parents may disagree about the best approach for managing the child's eating behaviors. In this scenario, the child is likely to align with whichever parent best supports the child's views, creating a triangle. Furthermore, in dysfunctional families, such as one in which a child is seriously overeating, members are overly emotionally reactive to each other. This extreme emotional reactivity perpetuates the cycle of overeating, because parents are likely to give into the child's protests against lifestyle changes. Finally, conflict between parents can lead to overfocus on the child, via the family projection process. When this occurs, one parent may overindulge the child's desires for food, continuing the cycle of unhealthy eating and obesity (Kaplan et al., 2014).

As demonstrated in the model above, principles from Bowen's family systems perspective can be applied to eating behaviors. This model could also be applied to families in which a child has an eating disorder. Consider a child living with symptoms of anorexia nervosa. That child's symptoms may cause parents to become highly anxious and overinvolved, leading to emotional fusion and overfunctioning on the part of one or both parents. The child, in turn, may become the focal point of the family's emotional process, representing the family projection process in which parental anxieties are unconsciously transmitted to the child. Triangulation can also develop, with one parent aligning with the child in support of their food refusal, while the other parent takes an opposing stance, deepening family conflict. Additionally, if the family has low levels of differentiation, emotional boundaries may become blurred, making it difficult for the child to develop autonomy and a stable identity. Thus, the systemic patterns described by Bowen may help clinicians understand how family anxiety and relational dynamics reinforce eating disorder symptoms (Brown & Errington, 2024).

In the aforementioned scenario, the child with anorexia nervosa becomes the family "symptom bearer," likely as a result of the family projection process, in which parents' anxieties are transmitted to the child. In cases of anorexia, the family anxiety manifests as rigid control of food intake and body weight. In an emotionally fused family, rigid control over food and body weight can also serve as a method to obtain some semblance of autonomy. So, the aim of family therapy would be to help family members establish higher levels of differentiation, rather than projecting anxieties onto the child and remaining emotionally fused (Brown & Errington, 2024).

Structural Family Therapy

Structural family therapy, the brainchild of Salvador Minuchin, is also among the family-focused interventions. This model agrees with Bowen's family systems perspective, in the sense that it views individual pathology not as a personal problem but rather as a problem that arises due to dysfunction within the larger family system. More specifically, according to the theory underlying structural family therapy, individual pathology occurs because of flawed organization of the family structure. The aim of structural family therapy is to restructure the family so family members can relate to each other in more adaptive ways (Wetchler & Hecker, 2015). The key assumptions of structural family therapy are described below.

Family Structure and Alliances

Structural family therapy views families as organizational systems with their own interaction patterns that determine how family members function. In families experiencing psychological distress, problems are viewed as being maintained by dysfunctional patterns of interaction. The structural family therapist is interested in how families organize themselves to resolve problems. Family organization refers to roles and power dynamics in families, including who is in charge and who takes on specific responsibilities. In families with flawed organization, some family members may form secret alliances with others, rather than directly addressing problems. Families may also perpetuate their own problems by intruding on one member's attempts to resolve the problem. While flawed family structure is seen as maintaining family problems, Minuchin was careful to avoid blaming families for their problems. Instead, he viewed families as being competent and simply requiring guidance to do away with dysfunctional structures (Wetchler & Hecker, 2015).

The Role of Boundaries

Boundaries are a central concept in structural family therapy, and they are closely related to subsystems, which are groupings of family members that unite for a specific task, role, or purpose. For instance, the parental subsystem involves the unity of mother and father for the purpose of nurturing, caring for, and disciplining children. Within families, boundaries define who is part of– as well as who isn't part of– a certain subsystem. Clear, healthy boundaries allow a subsystem to exist autonomously as a separate unit, but they also allow for contact with, rather than disengagement from, other subsystems in the family. On the other hand, enmeshed boundaries result in overinvolvement, leaving individuals and subsystems with little autonomy. This causes children to be drawn into marital problems and leaves family members without a sense of self. Alternatively, some dysfunctionally organized families have disengaged boundaries, in which individuals and subsystems are entirely closed off from outside interaction. In extreme cases, disengaged boundaries may result in parents knowing few to no details about their children's lives (Wetchler & Hecker, 2015).

Family Hierarchy

The family hierarchy is also central to structural family therapy. In healthy families, someone must assume leadership, and family leaders assume more power and decision-making responsibility than other members of the family. A specific hierarchy within a family is the parent-child hierarchy, which denotes the boundary between parental responsibilities and the role of the child. Family hierarchies become dysfunctional when parents do not have enough decision-making authority and thus cannot establish family rules or discipline children for misbehavior, (Wetchler & Hecker, 2015).

Coalitions

In structural family therapy, coalitions refer to a dynamic in which at least two family members come together against at least one other family member. This typically occurs in the context of two family members being in conflict, so the weaker member pulls in a third family member to support their viewpoint. Coalitions are typically hostile and secretive, and they prevent family problems from being resolved directly. Sometimes coalitions can be cross-generational, typically involving one spouse pulling a parent into conflict with the other spouse. These coalitions can also involve a parent pulling a child into conflict with the other parent. In a specific type of coalition called detouring, the parents avoid their own conflict by fixating on the child, thus resulting in the child becoming the problem, (Wetchler & Hecker, 2015).

The Process of Structural Family Therapy

The goal of structural family therapy is to help family members alter their structure to effectively resolve problems. Therapists using this modality must engage in a process called joining, whereby they communicate that they understand the family and desire to help. They must also engage in accommodation, which involves adapting one's actions to suit the needs of a specific family. After the therapist has engaged in joining and accommodation, they complete the process of structural diagnosis, which involves conducting assessment to identify what elements of family structure are dysfunctional. This assessment process tends to occur over multiple sessions through observation and interaction with families. Questions asked during the assessment process involve inquiries such as who makes decisions in the family, which family members are close to each other, and how parents differ in their discipline style. The therapist may also observe whether one child sits closer to one parent over the other, which may indicate a coalition (Wetchler & Hecker, 2015).

After assessment is complete, the structural family therapist works toward restructuring, or working with the family to create a better effective family structure. One tool used in the restructuring process is enactment, in which family members act out problems in the therapy session by discussing among themselves how to solve the problem. The therapist can then intervene by blocking unhelpful behaviors. For instance, if parents become distracted by the "problem child" during the session, the therapist may ask them to ignore that behavior and instead discuss between the two of them how to best assist the child. Other tools include boundary marking, in which the therapist helps families to create new boundaries, and unbalancing, in which the therapist temporarily aligns with the weaker family member to correct power imbalances (Wetchler & Hecker, 2015).

Structural Family Therapy for Eating Disorders

Structural family therapy has a role in eating disorder treatment; in some instances, the family structure may be ineffective for allowing parents to collaborate to address disordered eating. So, restructuring the family can promote problem resolution (Wetchler & Hecker, 2015). Some researchers have identified that families in which one member has an eating disorder tend to have a different structure from families in which there isn't a member with an eating disorder. More specifically, these families are more likely to have a poorly defined hierarchy and leadership system. These families also demonstrate dysfunctional patterns such as unpredictable rules, intergenerational coalitions, and distant or confrontational relationships between parents. Parents in these families also tend to have unrealistic or demanding expectations of their children (Mateos-Agut, et al., 2014). Based on this finding, some families in which a child has an eating disorder may benefit from the restructuring that structural family therapy offers.

Strategic Family Therapy

Strategic Family Therapy, including key approaches developed by Jay Haley, Cloé Madanes, and the MRI group, centers on identifying repetitive interaction patterns that sustain a family's presenting problem and then strategically interrupting those patterns through purposeful therapist interventions. Wetchler and Hecker (2015) explain that strategic therapists take an active and directive stance, which requires designing specific tasks or "directives" to break dysfunctional cycles and encourage immediate change in behavior or relational dynamics. A classic example is assigning a family member a paradoxical directive, in which the therapist tells the family to continue their problem behavior or perhaps even engage in the behavior more intensely. This sort of directive, though counterintuitive, can disrupt dysfunctional patterns (Wetchler & Hecker, 2015).

There are a variety of paradoxical directives or interventions in the strategic family therapy method. Strategic family therapists may use a technique called restraining change, which is a paradoxical intervention that encourages families to move slowly toward change. This can reduce the urgency associated with the problem and encourage families to comply with therapist's directives. Another paradoxical intervention involves prescribing the symptom, which involves telling the family to continue having the problem, with a goal of altering family interaction patterns and hierarchies (Wetchler & Hecker, 2015).

In families in which the therapist believes they have sufficient power for gaining compliance from family members, they may instead give straightforward directives, such as advice, suggestions, or information. These directives may involve coaching that helps parents to more effectively manage children or establish rules and consequences (Wetchler & Hecker, 2015).

Like family systems therapy, there is a paucity of literature directly analyzing strategic family therapy for the treatment of eating disorders. However, researchers have developed clinical protocols that utilize strategic family therapy in eating disorder treatment. For instance, Pietrabissa et al. (2019) have proposed the use of brief strategic therapy for treating bulimia nervosa and binge-eating disorder. Their protocol involves the prescription of a paradoxical diet, which directs the individual with the eating disorder to prepare the food they'd most like to eat and then eat as much of it as they desire. Patients may also be directed to regularly break their food rules and consume foods they would otherwise not allow themselves to have. For patients with bulimia, family members may be directed to ask a patient for a list of foods they'd like to vomit (Pietrabissa et al., 2019). These paradoxical directives serve the purpose of ridding the patient of temptation and breaking dysfunctional patterns.

Emotion-Focused Therapy

Principles from emotion-focused therapy may be integrated into family-based eating disorder treatments. In this model, parents serve as emotion coaches who help children identify, express, and regulate emotions. This model responds to the observation that parents' emotional blocks—such as fear, guilt, or self-blame—can interfere with effective caregiving in eating disorder recovery. By guiding parents to process their emotional responses, emotion-focused family therapy aims to strengthen their capacity to support their child's refeeding and symptoms in a calm manner (Goldman, 2019; Robinson et al., 2015).

Emotion-focused family therapy for eating disorders occurs in several phases. In the first phase, the parents and child receive education about emotions, including psychoeducation on the role that an eating disorder plays in avoiding or managing emotions. The parents learn to become emotion coaches, by identifying and responding to signs of emotion so they can better meet the child's emotional needs. As the family moves into the second phase of treatment, the parents become more independent in their roles as emotion coaches for the child. Parents can practice their skills at home, while also developing deeper empathy for the child during therapy sessions. This increased empathy will enhance the child's level of trust, resulting in the child becoming more comfortable sharing their emotional pain with parents. As time goes on, the child will no longer need to use disordered eating behaviors to manage painful emotions. During this second phase of treatment, the therapist also supports the parents in addressing any trauma the child has experienced. In the final phase of treatment, the child and parents can collaborate regarding the experience of emotion, with less and less support from the therapist. This allows the child to continue on a healthy developmental trajectory (Lafrance Robinson et al., 2015).

Potential Limitations Associated with Family-Based Therapy

There is evidence supporting the use of family interventions, especially for treating adolescents with anorexia nervosa. In fact, family-based treatment is considered the first choice for this population. Regardless, family-based models are not without limitations. One limitation is that clinicians tend to have misconceptions about this modality; therefore, they do not use it often in community-based settings. For instance, clinicians may have reservations about the effectiveness of family-based treatments and may find this modality to be difficult to implement with families. So, while family-based models may be the gold standard, it can be challenging to find a clinician who offers this type of treatment. Additional training for clinicians may be necessary to increase their comfort with offering family-based interventions so that patients and families can access this evidence-based treatment (Astrachan-Fletcher et al., 2018). Other research has revealed some barriers associated with family-based treatment, including lack of buy-in from caregivers of those with eating disorders, as well as challenges related to the time and resources required for families to participate in treatment (Gioia et al., 2025).

CONCLUSION

Family-focused treatment modalities have a place in eating disorder treatment, especially for children and adolescents. For adolescents with anorexia nervosa, Maudsley Family Therapy, also called manualized family-based treatment (FBT), appears to be the treatment of choice, but this modality may also play a role in treating adolescent bulimia nervosa (Brockmeyer et al., 2018; Loeb & le Grange, 2009). For some families, family systems therapy, with roots in Bowen's theory, may be effective for treating eating disorder symptoms in a child (Agras et al., 2014; Rockwell et al., 2011).

There is also some suggestion that the structural dysfunction in families who have a child with an eating disorder may benefit from structural family therapy (Mateos-Agut et al., 2014). In addition, the paradoxical interventions in strategic family therapy may break dysfunctional cycles that occur in eating disorders (Pietrabiassa et al., 2019), while emotion-focused family therapy can alleviate eating disorder symptoms in families in which children's emotional needs have historically been unmet (Lafrance Robinson et al., 2015) Regardless of the specific modality used, there is convincing evidence that family-focused treatments play a key role in the management of eating disorders in adolescent populations. Nonetheless, clinicians must consider the time and resources required for families to participate in treatment and make an effort to fully engage caregivers in the process (Gioia et al., 2025). Given time constraints, traditional family-based methods may require modifications to increase their feasibility.

REFERENCES

Agras, W. S., Lock, J., Brandt, H., Bryson, S. W., Dodge, E., Halmi, K. A., Jo, B., Johnson, C., Kaye, W., Wilfley, D., & Woodside, B. (2014). Comparison of 2 family therapies for adolescent anorexia nervosa: A randomized parallel trial. *JAMA Psychiatry*, *71*(11), 1279–1286. DOI: 10.1001/jamapsychiatry.2014.1025 PMID: 25250660

Astrachan-Fletcher, E., Accurso, E. C., Rossman, S., McClanahan, S. F., Dimitropoulos, G., & Le Grange, D. (2018). An exploratory study of challenges and successes in implementing adapted family-based treatment in a community setting. *Journal of Eating Disorders*, *6*(44), 44. Advance online publication. DOI: 10.1186/s40337-018-0228-9 PMID: 30603086

Brockmeyer, T., Friederich, H. C., & Schmidt, U. (2018). Advances in the treatment of anorexia nervosa: A review of established and emerging interventions. *Psychological Medicine*, *48*(8), 1228–1256. DOI: 10.1017/S0033291717002604 PMID: 28889819

Brown, J., & Errington, L. (2024). Bowen family systems theory and practice: Illustration and critique revisited. *Australian and New Zealand Journal of Family Therapy*, *45*(2), 135–155. DOI: 10.1002/anzf.1589

Calatrava, M., Martins, M. V., Schweer-Collins, M., Duch-Ceballos, C., & Rodríguez-González, M. (2022). Differentiation of self: A scoping review of Bowen Family Systems Theory's core construct. *Clinical Psychology Review*, *91*, 102101. Advance online publication. DOI: 10.1016/j.cpr.2021.102101 PMID: 34823190

Gioia, A. N., Morales, C., Laboe, A. A., Dolan, S. C., & Reilly, E. E. (2025). Clinical experiences using family based treatment for eating disorders. *International Journal of Eating Disorders*, *58*(4), 735–747. DOI: 10.1002/eat.24373 PMID: 39834197

Goldman, R. N. (2019). History and overview of emotion-focused therapy. In L. S. DOI: 10.1037/0000112-001

Jewell, T., Blessitt, E., Stewart, C., Simic, M., & Eisler, I. (2016). Family therapy for child and adolescent eating disorders: A critical review. *Family Process*, *55*(3), 577–594. DOI: 10.1111/famp.12242 PMID: 27543373

Kaplan, S. G., Arnold, E. M., Irby, M. B., Boles, K. A., & Skelton, J. A. (2014). Family systems theory and obesity treatment: Applications for clinicians. *Infant, Child & Adolescent Nutrition*, *6*(1), 24–29. DOI: 10.1177/1941406413516001 PMID: 24729831

Lafrance Robinson, A., Dolhanty, J., & Greenberg, L. (2015). Emotion-focused family therapy for eating disorders in children and adolescents. *Clinical Psychology & Psychotherapy*, *22*(1), 75–82. DOI: 10.1002/cpp.1861 PMID: 23913713

Lavender, K. R. (2020). Rebooting "failed" family-based treatment. *Frontiers in Psychiatry*, *11*(68), 68. Advance online publication. DOI: 10.3389/fpsyt.2020.00068 PMID: 32194444

Loeb, K. L., & Le Grange, D. (2009). Family-based treatment for adolescent eating disorders: Current status, new applications and future directions. *International Journal of Child and Adolescent Health*, *2*(2), 243–254. DOI: 10.1080/10640266.2010.509688 PMID: 20191109

Mateos-Agut, M., García-Alonso, I., De la Gándara-Martín, J. J., Vegas-Miguel, M. I., Sebastián-Vega, C., Sanz-Cid, B., Martínez-Villares, A., & Martín-Martínez, E. (2014). Family structure and eating behavior disorders. *Actas Españolas de Psiquiatría*, *42*(6), 267–280. https://actaspsiquiatria.es/index.php/actas/article/view/865 PMID: 25388769

Palombi, M. (2016). Separations: A personal account of Bowen Family Systems Theory. *Australian and New Zealand Journal of Family Therapy*, *37*(3), 327–339. DOI: 10.1002/anzf.1170

Pietrabissa, G., Castelnuovo, G., Jackson, J. B., Rossi, A., Manzoni, G. M., & Gibson, P. (2019). Brief strategic therapy for bulimia nervosa and binge eating disorder: A clinical and research protocol. *Frontiers in Psychology*, *10*, 373. DOI: 10.3389/fpsyg.2019.00373 PMID: 30906269

Rockwell, R. E., Boutelle, K., Trunko, M. E., Jacobs, M. J., & Kaye, W. H. (2011). An innovative short-term, intensive, family-based treatment for adolescent anorexia nervosa: Case series. *European Eating Disorders Review*, *19*(4), 362–367. DOI: 10.1002/erv.1094 PMID: 21308869

Wetchler, J. L., & Hecker, L. L. (2015). *An introduction to marriage and family therapy* (2nd ed.). Routledge.

KEY TERMS AND DEFINITIONS

Boundaries: A core concept in structural family therapy that refers to the rules that define who is and is not part of a family subsystem

Coalition: A term from structural family therapy that describes a dynamic in which two family members come together against another family member

Differentiation of Self: A core concept in Bowen's family systems therapy, which refers to a person's ability to remain both connected independent

Emotional Cut-Off: A process in which a person distances themselves, either emotionally or physically, from their family of origin in order to cope with intense fusion

Emotion-Focused Therapy: A modality used in eating disorder treatment that involves teaching parents to appropriately support their child's emotional needs

Family Hierarchy: The structure in families that determines who assumes a leadership role

Family Projection Process: A process in which parents focus intensely on one child in the family, thereby projecting their own problems onto the child

Family Systems Therapy: A therapy modality based on the work of Murray Bowen, who viewed families as interconnected emotional systems

Multigenerational Transmission Process: The tendency for differentiation to be passed down from one generation to the next, causing family problems that persist across generations

Nuclear Family Emotional System: The pattern of emotional functioning within a family

Paradoxical Directives: Interventions in strategic therapy that involve counterintuitive instructions, such as telling a family to engage in the problem behavior

Strategic Family Therapy: A treatment modality that focuses on interrupting interaction patterns that sustain a family's problem by using purposeful interventions

Structural Family Therapy: A treatment modality that emphasizes reorganizing families to better equip them to solve problems

The Maudsley Method: A family-based eating disorder treatment method, also called manualized family-based treatment, in which the initial phase of treatment involves a parent taking control of the ill child's eating habits

Triangles: A process in which two people are in conflict and a third party is pulled into the dynamic to reduce the tension

Chapter 10
Group-Based Interventions for Eating Disorders

ABSTRACT

This chapter provides an overview of group-based interventions for eating disorders. It begins with an overview of the benefits of group treatments and then discusses the stages of group. Then, the chapter discusses specific group treatment modalities, such as cognitive-behavioral groups, DBT skills groups, psychoeducation groups, parenting groups, and psychodynamic groups. The evidence base supporting each group modality is also discussed. The chapter concludes with a list of recommended further reading.

INTRODUCTION

Previous chapters have described both individual and family-focused eating disorder treatment modalities, but a textbook on evidence-based eating disorder treatments would be incomplete without a discussion of group-based modalities. Meta-analytic research has revealed that group-based interventions are effective for treating binge-eating disorder (O'Connor et al., 2024). An earlier meta-analysis also found that group psychotherapy was superior to a waitlist control condition for treating binge-eating and purging symptoms (Grenon et al., 2017). Additionally, group cognitive behavioral therapy has been identified as effective for

DOI 10.4018/979-8-3373-0664-3.ch010

reducing perfectionism in individuals with anorexia nervosa (Lloyd et al., 2014). Given the evidence base supporting group-based eating disorder interventions, it is essential for current and future clinicians to have foundational knowledge of this treatment modality. This chapter describes group-based interventions for eating disorders, beginning with an overview of the process of group therapy, and progressing to a discussion of specific group interventions.

THE FOUNDATIONS OF GROUP THERAPY

There are various types of group therapy, each with its own theoretical orientation. However, there are some features that tend to be consistent across the group therapy modalities. Most groups used in eating disorder treatment fall under the category of a psychotherapy group, which seeks to assist people with overcoming psychological problems. People participating in psychotherapy groups usually have a mental health diagnosis that causes significant distress and interferes with their daily functioning. Some eating disorder groups may fall under the umbrella of a psychoeducational group, which provides members with essential information about eating disorder symptoms (Corey et al., 2018).

Regardless of the specific theoretical orientation of the group, patients tend to benefit from a range of therapeutic factors that are specific to the group modality. For example, cohesion among group members is considered to be a therapeutic factor, as it's linked to patient improvement. Cohesion is also associated with a sense of trust and support within a group, which can benefit patients, regardless of the specific theory guiding the group. Other therapeutic factors associated with group include forming a therapeutic alliance with the group leader, having an opportunity to express emotions, and gaining deeper understanding of one's own problems. Finally, participating in a group is associated with the concept of universality, as it helps members to recognize that they are not alone, as others are experiencing similar problems (Landi et al., 2021). The bottom line is that group therapy comes with unique benefits related to the process of participating in a group, in addition to exposing members to a particular therapeutic modality.

Stages of Group Therapy

There are multiple different stage models of group therapy, but what they all have in common is the belief that when people come together to participate in a group, the work unfolds in stages. In the initial stages of group, members are becoming oriented to the group, and they tend to be cautious about what they share with other group members. They may have anxiety about sharing personal problems with other group members, and it's essential for the group leader to create a safe environment. Before progressing into deeper work within the group therapy setting, members must also endure the transition stage, during which some members may be defensive and fearful of sharing. During the transition stage, there is a tension between remaining safe by not sharing and taking the risks associated with opening up to others. Group leaders should not force members to share but instead should respect members' fears. After progressing through the transition stage of group, members are ready to enter the working stage, which involves group members committing to thoroughly explore their presenting problems with the group. In a working group, there is an environment of trust among members, and people openly share with others, in addition to offering feedback. During the final stage of group, members work toward termination and discuss how they will take what they have learned in group and maintain it in daily life (Corey et al., 2018). Some stage models may utilize different terms to describe each stage, but most theories of group development posit that members must undergo a process of orienting to the group and developing a sense of trust or safety before moving into deeper therapeutic work. The group leader plays an important role in creating that sense of trust and safety and must be prepared to support members as the group develops through various stages.

SPECIFIC GROUP THERAPY MODALITIES

Group therapy, as its name suggests, involves participating in therapeutic services in a group setting, with others experiencing similar challenges. While all groups tend to offer therapeutic benefits, such as cohesion with other members, there are multiple different types of group therapy, all with their own theoretical orientation. The different types of therapy groups utilized in eating disorder treatment are detailed below.

Psychoeducation Groups

Psychoeducation groups are designed to provide education to participants to help them cope with whatever problem has brought them to the group. In the case of psychoeducation groups for eating disorders, this might involve learning about symptoms, risk factors, and consequences of eating disorders, in addition to learning coping skills. Researchers recently evaluated the effects of a group psychoeducation treatment for individuals with binge-eating disorder. Participants attended one 90-minute session per week for 12 weeks, and 6-11 people with an average age of around 47 years, participated in each group. The program began with eight teaching modules led by a psychiatry resident and a clinical psychologist. During the second part of treatment, a dietician worked with the mental health providers to provide health education lessons (Liquori et al., 2022).

The first session of the aforementioned program emphasized the use of a food diary in which group members recorded their daily food intake as well as their emotions, thoughts, and level of hunger or fullness when eating. Participants were instructed on how to use the food diary; they also received education related to the definition of binge-eating. During later education sessions, participants learned about the impact of emotion regulation on binge-eating and the role that interpersonal stressors can play in the disorder. Health education sessions provided information about macronutrients, how to shop for groceries, and how to make lifestyle changes to reduce binge-eating. At the end of the study, data analysis found that those who participated in the group showed reductions and body mass index and binge-eating; they also showed an improvement in their own body image (Liquori et al. 2022).

The group modality described above was effective for reducing problems related to binge-eating disorder, and this result is in agreement with the larger body of research related to psychoeducation groups for eating disorders. One recent meta-analysis which reviewed the results of psychoeducation programs, many of which were delivered in group format, found that these programs were effective for treating eating disorders, because they led to weight gain and a decrease in symptoms. These programs involved those delivered to children, adolescents, and caregivers; those delivered to caregivers resulted in a reduction in the burden placed on the caregivers (Kurnik Mesarič et al., 2024). This finding demonstrates that psychoeducation groups are also beneficial for children and their families.

Cognitive-Behavioral Groups

Individual cognitive-behavioral therapy (CBT) was discussed earlier in its own chapter, but this modality can also be delivered in a group format. Research has evaluated the benefits of group CBT for treating binge-eating disorder. In one protocol, individuals with binge-eating disorder participated in 20 hour-long group BT sessions. The beginning sessions emphasized the use of daily self-monitoring to normalize eating patterns, and then middle sessions focused on cognitive restructuring to change thought patterns linked to binge-eating. Finally, the last six sessions taught relapse prevention skills, such as problem-solving and coping with triggers. Study results revealed that group CBT was just as effective as individual CBT for reducing binge-eating and body weight (Ricca et al., 2010).

Researchers have also evaluated the effects of group cognitive behavioral therapy for patients with anorexia nervosa. One group intervention rooted in CBT targeted distorted thinking related to perfectionism to enable group members to develop more manageable standards for themselves. The group was carried out in an inpatient treatment setting with four to seven members per group. The group intervention involved six hour-long sessions. At the end of group, members showed significant improvements in perfectionism, which is promising, since this personality trait is linked to a maintenance of eating disorder symptoms. Participants also found the group to be helpful for gaining insight into the problems associated with perfectionism (Lloyd et al., 2014). This study provides additional support for the use of group CBT interventions in eating disorder treatment.

Psychodynamic Group Therapy

There is some evidence that psychodynamic group therapy can be effective for reducing eating disorder symptoms. However, existing research using the psychodynamic method often does not use manualized treatments, and some studies use psychodynamic therapy in combination with other therapeutic orientations, such as CBT. It can therefore be challenging to separate benefits of psychodynamic group therapy from those of other modalities. Nonetheless, existing research does suggest that psychodynamic group treatment can lead to improvement in some eating disorder symptoms (Trombetta et al., 2024).

The existing research shows that psychodynamic group therapies are most effective for patients with bulimia nervosa and binge-eating disorder, while results are not as promising for those with anorexia nervosa. There are mixed results related to group psychodynamic treatment of anorexia. Generally speaking, the group psychodynamic modalities explore defense mechanisms, unconscious conflict, internalized object relations, and the influence of past experiences (Trombetta et al., 2024). Research has found group modalities incorporating psychodynamic and interpersonal therapy to be especially effective for reducing binge-eating. One study that yielded promising results with group psychodynamic/interpersonal therapy treated binge-eating as a way to cope with the uncomfortable emotions associated with unmet attachment needs. This intervention also operated according to the belief that past attachment issues manifest as dysfunctional interpersonal patterns in the present, which perpetuates the cycle of binge-eating to cope with negative emotions. In the group setting, dysfunctional interpersonal interaction patterns reveal themselves, and members have the opportunity to practice more adaptive interactions with other group members (O'Connor et al., 2024).

DBT Skills Groups

As discussed in an earlier chapter, there is evidence supporting the use of DBT in eating disorders treatment (Brown et al., 2020). Group-based skills training is a core component of DBT, teaching mindfulness, emotion regulation, distress tolerance, and interpersonal effectiveness (Linehan &

Wilks, 2015). Some authors have evaluated the use of DBT interventions that utilize only the group skills training component for the treatment of eating disorders. For example, one study used Linehan's original DBT treatment manual to create an adapted version of DBT consisting of 20 group-based skills sessions. Sessions were held weekly for two hours. The mindfulness component of this treatment modality taught participants to develop present-moment awareness of their emotions by describing them and allowing them to pass without judgment, which puts a stop to the cycle of binge-eating to avoid uncomfortable emotions. After learning mindfulness skills, participants progressed to learning emotion regulation, which allowed them to identify emotional states that tend to trigger binges and notice bodily sensations linked to such emotions. In the final stages of the group DBT modality, participants learned distress tolerance skills, like distracting themselves with a walk or soothing themselves with a warm bath, rather than turning to binge-eating to manage stress. At the end of the treatment, 82% of the women in the study were no longer binge-eating (Telch et al., 2000).

A more recent study evaluated the effects of a DBT skills group used as an add-on to family-based treatment for adolescents with anorexia nervosa or other restrictive eating behaviors. Participants engaged in a DBT skills group once per week for 6 months. The treatment resulted in reductions in binge-eating and maladaptive coping strategies coupled with increases in weight gain. This study provides preliminary evidence supporting DBT skills groups in the treatment of anorexia nervosa (Peterson et al. 2020).

Parent Groups

Parents of children and adolescents living with eating disorders may participate in group skills training with other parents. One parent skills training modality, based on the New Maudsley treatment approach, offered 14 hours of group training to parents over the course of two consecutive days. The group training program required parents to read two chapters from a book on caring for people with eating disorders. During the training program, parents received educational programming in addition to participating in group discussions and role-playing activities and watching therapists modeling skills. Based on qualitative analysis, this program was beneficial for increasing parent self-efficacy while improving psychological distress, anxiety, and caregiver burden (Goodier et al., 2014). Parents who participate in skills training may find themselves better prepared to manage their child's eating disorder, as well as less distressed by the caregiving experience.

Some parents of children with eating disorders may benefit from participating in support groups to help them cope with the stressors associated with caring for a child with an eating disorder. With recent technological advances, support groups may be delivered online, making them easily accessible. One recent study evaluated the benefits of a virtual peer support group offered to parents of children with eating disorders. Group facilitators were parents who had lived experience with caring for a child who had recovered from an eating disorder. Support group meetings offered education on relevant topics, as well as opportunities to hear from guest speakers. Qualitative data analysis revealed that participants benefited from learning about eating disorders, offering support to others, and connecting with those experiencing similar challenges. Support groups may offer parents a means of coping with their child's eating disorder, thereby making them more effective as caretakers (Grennan et al., 2022).

LIMITATIONS OF GROUP THERAPY

There is evidence, including from meta-analytic research, that group interventions are effective for treating eating disorders (Grenon et al., 2017; Kurnik Mesarič et al., 2024; O'Connor et al., 2024). There isn't as much research supporting group therapy for anorexia nervosa and bulimia nervosa when compared to binge-eating disorder, so more research is needed. In the meantime, clinicians should use caution when referring patients with anorexia nervosa or bulimia nervosa to group treatment, engaging in careful evaluation to ensure patient progress for those referred to group therapy. Patients with anorexia or bulimia diagnoses should also be informed of the lack of evidence evaluating group treatment for their respective diagnoses (O'Connor et al., 2024).

CONCLUSION

There are drawbacks associated with group therapy, primarily related to the lack of research supporting its use with those living with anorexia and bulimia. Nonetheless, clinicians working in the arena of eating disorder treatment may run therapy groups as a part of patient care. In this case, they must be prepared to develop a therapeutic alliance with participants and create a sense of safety within the group, allowing participants time to develop trust in the group (Corey et al., 2018; Landi et al., 2021). Even if clinicians do not directly run therapy groups, they may determine that a particular patient would benefit from group therapy, warranting a referral for such services. Regardless of the role a professional plays in relationship to group therapy, it's essential for practitioners to be aware of group treatment modalities for eating disorders. Those preparing to deliver group interventions should review treatment protocol manuals and ensure they develop training and competence in the specific group modality they are delivering. For those interested in developing competence in specific group therapy methods, the list of additional readings at the end of this chapter may be of interest.

REFERENCES

Brown, T. A., Wisniewski, L., & Anderson, L. K. (2020). Dialectical behavior therapy for eating disorders: State of the research and new directions. *Eating Disorders*, *28*(2), 97–100. DOI: 10.1080/10640266.2020.1728204 PMID: 32301685

Corey, M., Corey, G., & Corey, C. (2018). *Groups: Process and practice* (10th ed.). Cengage.

Goodier, G. H. G., McCormack, J., Egan, S. J., Watson, H. J., Hoiles, K. J., & Byrne, S. M. (2014). Parent skills training treatment for parents of children and adolescents with eating disorders: A qualitative study. *International Journal of Eating Disorders*, *47*(4), 368–375. DOI: 10.1002/eat.22224 PMID: 24843891

Grennan, L., Nicula, M., Pellegrini, D., Giuliani, K., Crews, E., Webb, C., Gouveia, M.-R., Loewen, T., & Couturier, J. (2022). "I'm not alone": A qualitative report of experiences among parents of children with eating disorders attending virtual parent-led peer support groups. *Journal of Eating Disorders*, *10*(195), 195. Advance online publication. DOI: 10.1186/s40337-022-00719-2 PMID: 36522772

Grenon, R., Schwartze, D., Hammond, N., Ivanova, I., Mcquaid, N., Proulx, G., & Tasca, G. A. (2017). Group psychotherapy for eating disorders: A meta-analysis. *International Journal of Eating Disorders*, *50*(9), 997–1013. DOI: 10.1002/eat.22744 PMID: 28771758

Kurnik Mesarič, K., Damjanac, Ž., Debeljak, T., & Kodrič, J. (2024). Effectiveness of psychoeducation for children, adolescents and caregivers in the treatment of eating disorders: A systematic review. *European Eating Disorders Review*, *32*(1), 99–115. DOI: 10.1002/erv.3028 PMID: 37656835

Landi, G., Simoni, E., Landi, I., Galeazzi, G. M., Moscara, M., Pighi, M., & Di Lorenzo, R. (2021). Therapeutic factors in a psychiatric group therapy: A preliminary validation of Therapeutic Factors Inventory-8, Italian version. *The Psychiatric Quarterly*, *92*(2), 523–536.

Linehan, M. M., & Wilks, C. R. (2015). The course and evolution of dialectical behavior therapy. *American Journal of Psychotherapy*, *69*(2), 97–110. DOI: 10.1176/appi.psychotherapy.2015.69.2.97 PMID: 26160617

Liquori, S., Faidutti, G., Garzitto, M., Saetti, L., Bendotti, M., & Balestrieri, M. (2022). Efficacy of a group psychoeducation treatment in binge eating disorder: An open-label study. *Frontiers in Psychiatry*, *13*, 822282. Advance online publication. DOI: 10.3389/fpsyt.2022.822282 PMID: 35558418

Lloyd, S., Fleming, C., Schmidt, U., & Tchanturia, K. (2014). Targeting perfectionism in anorexia nervosa using a group-based cognitive behavioural approach: A pilot study. *European Eating Disorders Review*, *22*(5), 366–372. DOI: 10.1002/erv.2313 PMID: 25113819

O'Connor, E., Garceau, C., Polhill, S., & Tasca, G. A. (2024). Evidence-based group therapy for eating disorders. *Group Dynamics*, *28*(3), 163–177. DOI: 10.1037/gdn0000221

Peterson, C. M., Kroon Van Diest, A. M., Mara, C. A., & Matthews, A. (2020). Dialectical behavioral therapy skills group as an adjunct to family-based therapy in adolescents with restrictive eating disorders. *Eating Disorders*, *28*(1), 67–79. DOI: 10.1080/10640266.2019.1568101 PMID: 30669955

Ricca, V., Castellini, G., Mannucci, E., Lo Sauro, C., Ravaldi, C., Rotella, C. M., & Faravelli, C. (2010). Comparison of individual and group cognitive behavioral therapy for binge eating disorder: A randomized, three-year follow-up study. *Appetite*, *55*(3), 656–665. DOI: 10.1016/j.appet.2010.09.019 PMID: 20870000

Telch, C. F., Agras, W. S., & Linehan, M. M. (2000). Group dialectical behavior therapy for binge-eating disorder: A preliminary, uncontrolled trial. *Behavior Therapy*, *31*(3), 569–582. DOI: 10.1016/S0005-7894(00)80031-3

Trombetta, T., Bottaro, D., Paradiso, M. N., Santoniccolo, F., Abbate Daga, G., & Rollè, L. (2024). Psychodynamic group therapy for eating disorders: A narrative review. *Journal of Contemporary Psychotherapy*, *54*(3), 253–264. DOI: 10.1007/s10879-023-09614-6

ADDITIONAL READING

Karoll, C., & Silverman, A. (2024). *Eating disorder group therapy: A collaborative approach* (1st ed.). Routledge. DOI: 10.4324/9781003430964

Safer, D. L., Telch, C. F., & Chen, E. Y. (2017). *Dialectical behavior therapy for binge eating and bulimia* (Foreword by M. M. Linehan). Guilford Press

Tchanturia, K. (Ed.). (2015). *Brief group psychotherapy for eating disorders: Inpatient protocols*. Routledge. DOI: 10.4324/9781315720364

KEY TERMS AND DEFINITIONS

Cognitive Behavioral Group Therapy: A group treatment modality that emphasizes cognitive restructuring, correction of distorted thinking patterns, problem-solving, and relapse prevention

DBT Skills Group: A group treatment modality based on principles from Dialectical Behavior Therapy (DBT) that teaches skills for mindfulness, emotion regulation, distress tolerance, and interpersonal effectiveness

Psychodynamic Group Therapy: A group treatment modality that emphasizes the role of unconscious conflicts, internalized object relations, past experiences, and unmet attachment needs in the maintenance of eating disorder symptoms

Psychoeducation Group: A group treatment modality that emphasizes providing information to participants to improve their coping

Psychotherapy Group: A group treatment modality suitable for individuals who mental health problems that interfere with daily functioning and/or cause significant distress

Transition Stage: The phase of group therapy during which participants are torn between staying safe and taking risks, so they may show resistance towards sharing in group

Universality: A benefit imparted by group therapy that enables members to feel less alone, as they realize others share their struggles

Working Stage: The phase of group therapy during which group members are committed to solving problems and sharing openly in group

Section 3
Additional Considerations in Eating Disorder Treatment

Chapter 11
Level of Care in Eating Disorder Treatment

ABSTRACT

This chapter describes levels of care in eating disorder treatment, including inpatient, residential, partial hospitalization, intensive outpatient, and standard outpatient. Each level of care is discussed in detail. The chapter also provides guidance for assessing the appropriate level of care for each patient and concludes with professional guidelines for determining the most appropriate level of care for a given patient. Guidelines are based on standards from the American Psychiatric Association and Massachusetts General Hospital.

INTRODUCTION

The previous chapters in this text have described evidence-based interventions for eating disorders, covering individual, family-based, and group treatments. Also critical to effective eating disorder treatment is selecting an appropriate level of care for a patient's clinical presentation. Some patients may have a more severe clinical presentation, warranting a higher level of care, whereas others may be appropriate for less intensive outpatient treatment. It is essential for eating disorder clinicians to understand the different levels of care, as well as how to assess a patient to determine the appropriate level of care for beginning treatment. In the sections that follow, the different levels of care in eating disorder treatment

DOI 10.4018/979-8-3373-0664-3.ch011

are discussed, and readers are introduced to assessment tools that are useful for determining the appropriate level of care for a patient.

AVAILABLE LEVELS OF CARE

When a person seeks treatment for an eating disorder, there are various levels of care at which they may begin their treatment. Levels of care range from outpatient treatment, at the lowest level of care, all the way to inpatient hospitalization, which is the highest level of care (Anderson et al., 2017). The different levels of care are discussed below in more detail.

Inpatient Hospitalization

Inpatient hospitalization is the highest level of care, typically reserved for patients who are medically unstable. At this level of care, the patient has access to medical care around-the-clock, and staff supervise meals. For patients who require it, one-on-one supervision is typically available (Anderson et al., 2017). In some cases, patients may require involuntary hospitalization if the eating disorder is severe, and they refuse treatment. Should this be necessary, patients should be placed in a specialized eating disorder unit that provides access to multidisciplinary care, rather than a general psychiatric unit (Pehliven et al. 2022).

The nature of treatment provided in inpatient hospital settings can vary, based on a patient's diagnosis. For patients with anorexia nervosa, inpatient treatment emphasizes medical stabilization. Research has shown that inpatient hospitalization can contribute to weight gain and reduce symptoms related to anorexia; however, it may not confer additional benefits beyond outpatient care. Shorter stays in inpatient care are becoming the norm for the treatment of anorexia nervosa. In cases of bulimia nervosa, inpatient hospitalization is effective for reducing eating disorder symptoms and the severity of binging and purging. Inpatient care for bulimia tends to emphasize the provision of psychotherapy, and there is no indication that longer stays are linked to better outcomes (Pehliven et al., 2022).

For the treatment of avoidant/restrictive food intake disorder (ARFID), the goal of inpatient care is to restore weight and nutritional status. Evidence shows that inpatient care for ARFID is effective for increasing food intake post-discharge as well as for promoting weight gain. Patients diagnosed with ARFID tend to require longer courses of inpatient hospitalization when compared to those with an anorexia nervosa diagnosis; those with ARFID are also more likely to rely on tube feeding (Pehliven et al., 2022).

Residential Treatment

Just below inpatient hospitalization is the residential level of treatment. What differentiates residential treatment from inpatient hospitalization is the availability of medical services. A hospital is able to provide the highest level of medical care, including refeeding, which can occur via nasogastric tube in the hospital setting (Bendall & Taylor, 2023). Residential treatment centers are unlikely to offer tube feeding, but they provide multidisciplinary treatment in a home-like setting. Patients in residential treatment live on-site at a facility, while participating in individual and group therapy and recreational activities. They also receive meals on site, and staff provide support with maintaining stable eating patterns. Residential treatment is appropriate for patients who are medically stable and therefore do not require inpatient hospitalization, but who require a higher level of care than what can be provided in the outpatient setting (Peckmezian & Paxton, 2020). For instance, a patient who is at high risk of relapse may benefit from the structure that outpatient care provides. Fortunately, most research with residential treatment for eating disorders has yielded positive outcomes, including improvements to eating disorder symptoms, body weight, depression, and quality of life (Peckmezian & Paxton, 2020).

Partial Hospitalization Programming

Partial hospitalization programming (PHP) is at the step below residential treatment. Patients in a PHP attend treatment most days of the week in an outpatient setting, meaning they return home at night. A PHP offers services from 3 to 7 days a week, for between 6 to 10 hours a day.

The benefit of a PHP is that it allows patients to continue to live at home and practice recovery-related skills in daily life, but they have a higher level of structure than can be provided at lower levels of outpatient care. A PHP offers a range of services, such as individual and group therapy and consultation with a dietician and psychiatrist. Interestingly, some research suggests that a PHP is just as effective as inpatient care, and more effective than traditional outpatient programming. Furthermore, PHP is more cost-effective than inpatient and residential treatment options (Anderson et al., 2017).

Intensive Outpatient Programming

Intensive outpatient programming (IOP) is at a lower level of care than a PHP, but at a higher level than standard outpatient treatment. Individuals participating in IOP attend treatment at a clinic or other outpatient facility for around 3 hours per day for 3 to 5 days out of the week. Like PHP, IOP gives patients access to a range of services, including medication management, nutrition care, and both individual and group therapy (Anderson et al., 2017).

Standard Outpatient Programming

Finally, standard outpatient programming refers to any treatment modality that offers fewer than 9 hours of services per week. Patients in standard outpatient treatment may attend one hour-long therapy session per week, alongside a weekly support group, for example.

DETERMING THE MOST APPROPRIATE LEVEL OF CARE

Clinicians conducting an initial assessment of a patient's treatment needs will likely make a determination about the most appropriate level of care for that patient. There is not one straightforward manner to determine the best level of care for a particular patient (Anderson et al., 2017). However, the American Psychiatric Association (2023) offers practice guidelines for treating eating disorders, and these guidelines are useful when determining the most appropriate level of care for a patient's needs. Aside from the American Psychiatric Association, the Royal Australian and New Zealand College of Psychiatrists (RANZCP) and the National Institute of Clinical Excellence offer guidelines for determining level of care (Anderson et al., 2017). There is some overlap among these guidelines, which is discussed below.

When Inpatient Treatment is Most Appropriate

While inpatient care may not always offer additional benefits when compared to outpatient treatment (Pehliven et al., 2022), some patients require inpatient treatment for safety and stabilization. The three guidelines noted above all agree that a patient who is medically unstable should be placed in an inpatient treatment program (American Psychiatric Association, 2023; Anderson et al., 2017). Indicators of medical instability in adults include a heart rate below 40 beats per minute, blood pressure under 90/60 mmHG, blood glucose under 60 mg/DL, dehydration, poorly-functioning organs, low potassium levels, low body temperature, electrolyte imbalances, uncontrolled diabetes, and BMI below 14kg/m2. In pediatric patients, including adolescents, a heart rate near 40 beats per minute; low blood pressure; and low levels of phosphorus, potassium, or magnesium are considered indicative of medical instability (Anderson et al., 2017).

In addition to the criteria outlined above, some patients may require inpatient treatment if eating disorder symptoms, such as forced vomiting or laxative misuse, are uncontrolled and would benefit from around-the-clock supervision. A patient may also require inpatient treatment if they present with active suicidal ideation or severe self-harming behavior (American Psychiatric Association, 2023; Anderson et al., 2017). Finally, a patient who is resistant to treatment, who is in active psychosis, or who has not improved with outpatient care may benefit from inpatient services (American Psychiatric Association, 2023).

When Residential Treatment is Most Appropriate

Residential treatment is unlikely to be suitable for a patient who requires tube feeding (Bendall & Taylor, 2023), nor can it meet the acute needs of a patient who is medically unstable (American Psychiatric Association, 2023). However, some patients may require a higher level of care than outpatient treatment offers. For instance, the American Psychiatric Association (2023), states that patients who have co-occurring conditions, such as a substance use disorder, may require a higher level of care. Similarly, some patients may require monitoring to help them put a stop to behaviors like restrictive eating or purging; in this instance, residential care may be more suitable. Finally, a patient who has a stressful home environment could benefit from residential care, as this treatment setting removes the patient from stressors and allows them to focus solely on their recovery.

When Outpatient Treatment is Most Appropriate

There are various levels of outpatient care– PHP, IOP, and standard outpatient. PHP provides a structured environment with multiple hours of support per day. Some programs even offer treatment services 7 days per week. Since PHPs tend to be more cost-effective than inpatient treatment, these programs can be beneficial for patients who have complex needs, such as severe symptoms, co-occurring disorders, or the need for monitoring, but who cannot access inpatient or residential care due to financial barriers (Anderson et al., 2017).

Partial hospitalization programs can offer meal monitoring, as well as access to integrated services, including individual and group counseling, nutritional interventions, monitored meals, psychiatric care, and medical consultation. However, these programs do not have physicians and nursing staff on-site around-the-clock, and they cannot provide medical monitoring or tube feeding (American Psychiatric Association, 2023). So, this setting is appropriate for patients with complex needs, but not those who are medically fragile or in need of 24-hour-a-day supervision.

As a step-down from PHP, IOP does not offer as much monitoring and may not be the choice for patients with more complex treatment needs.

IOPs are typically able to monitor one meal per day, and they offer individual, group, and family counseling. These programs sometimes offer medication management, and they are an appropriate fit for individuals who prefer to work or attend school while in treatment (American Psychiatric Association, 2023).

Intensive outpatient care is appropriate in patients who are medically stable and not in need of a higher level of care due to malnutrition. It is also important for patients in outpatient treatment to be psychologically stable, and symptoms should not be so severe that they warrant a higher level of care with more consistent monitoring. Some research does suggest that outpatient programs providing cognitive-behavioral therapy specific to eating disorders (CBT-E) can be effective even in severe cases of anorexia nervosa. However, the patient must demonstrate motivation to participate in treatment; if the patient does not show weight gain and other indicators of positive response to outpatient treatment, entering a PHP, residential, or inpatient program is the next step (Frosstad & Bentz, 2022). According to a report by the National Eating Disorders Association (NEDA), a person must be able to function in daily life and apply skills learned during therapy to real-life settings to be successful with intensive outpatient treatment (Graves, n.d.).

Finally, outpatient treatment, at the lowest level of care, offers one to two therapy sessions per week. This level of care does not offer meal monitoring, so family members must be prepared to monitor meals, if indicated. There is limited access to physicians and other providers in standard outpatient treatment, so the patient must be able to access these providers at other facilities within the community if needed (American Psychiatric Association, 2023). Since standard outpatient treatment is the lowest level of care, it is typically a step-down from higher levels of care, such as intensive outpatient or PHP.

OTHER CONSIDERATIONS RELATED TO LEVEL OF CARE

The guidelines provided above are just that– guidelines. While they provide helpful information for providers making determinations regarding level of care, the reality is that selecting the best treatment setting for a patient may not always be black-and-white. Beyond the guidelines discussed above, there are additional factors that may affect decisions related to level of care.

For instance, some patients may require a higher level of care due to psychiatric concerns. To be appropriate for intensive outpatient treatment, a patient must show psychiatric stability. So, someone who is medically stable with symptoms not severe enough to require around-the-clock monitoring may require a higher level of care than intensive outpatient treatment if they have psychiatric comorbidities. Some individuals with co-occurring mental health disorders may present as psychiatrically stable but still require frequent monitoring of mental health symptoms. In this case, a PHP may be more appropriate than intensive outpatient services. On the other hand, a patient who is medically stable but has severe psychiatric symptoms may require residential treatment, so they have access to around-the-clock care (Graves, n.d.).

In patients with anorexia nervosa, comorbidities, including substance use disorders, personality disorders, autism spectrum disorder, depression, anxiety, and obsessive-compulsive disorder are common and can lead to a need for a higher level of care (Frostad & Bentz, 2022). One study found that 71% of individuals with eating disorders had at least one psychiatric comorbidity, and anxiety disorders were the most common co-occurring diagnosis. Men with bulimia and women with binge-eating disorder were most likely to have psychiatric comorbidities, according to study results (Ulfvebrand et al., 2015). Given the high prevalence of psychiatric comorbidities in patients with eating disorders, this is a critical consideration when determining the best placement for a particular patient.

Finally, individuals with lower body mass index (BMI) and previous residential treatment admission may require a higher level of care, or additional supportive services to prevent complications. Patients who present with one of these risk factors may benefit from treatment in a partial hospitalization setting, rather than intensive or standard outpatient services, to prevent hospitalization (Simpson et al., 2021).

ASSESSING FOR THE BEST LEVEL OF CARE

As indicated in the sections above, determining the most suitable level of care for a patient depends upon several factors, such as medical and psychiatric stability, psychological needs, symptom severity, body weight, and the extent to which a patient requires monitoring. Since there are not always straightforward criteria that determine the best level of care, selecting the most appropriate treatment setting for a patient can be challenging. Fortunately, the Massachusetts General Hospital (MGH) provides rather concise guidelines for determining the best level of care, based on medical status, suicidality, body weight, motivation, co-occurring disorders, environment stressors, need for structure, ability to control purging and excessive exercise, and proximity to treatment providers (Guarda & Schreyer, 2010).

Below are essential pieces from the MGH guidelines, which can be useful when making decisions related to level of care (Guarda & Schreyer 2010):

- Adults who are medically unstable, as evidenced by organ malfunction, low blood pressure or heart rate, low blood glucose, electrolyte imbalances, dehydration, or type 1 diabetes, require inpatient hospitalization. Children who are medically unstable also require inpatient hospitalization, but the definition of instability varies from that of adults.
- Patients who have a lethal suicide plan or who are otherwise at high risk of suicide are likely to require inpatient care.
- Patients who have a body weight above 85% of the expectation for their height and developmental level are generally appropriate for outpatient care, unless other factors suggest a higher level of care is warranted.
- Outpatient treatment is appropriate for those with fair-to-good motivation, whereas those with poor motivation are more appropriate for residential treatment or inpatient care.
- The presence of co-occurring psychiatric conditions is a key consideration when determining level of care.

- Individuals who are self-sufficient can be placed in outpatient or intensive outpatient care, whereas those who require structure to gain weight are more appropriate for partial hospitalization.
- Patients who will restrict food without supervision during meals require residential treatment, whereas those requiring tube feeding must be placed in inpatient care.
- Patients who have extreme family conflict or a lack of support at home may require a higher level of care.
- A patient's proximity to a treatment center must also be considered; outpatient treatment closer to home may be preferable to an inpatient or residential facility farther from home.
- Patients who can use self-control to prevent behaviors like purging or compulsive exercise in unstructured settings are appropriate for lower levels of care, whereas those who require structure and cannot prevent purging are more appropriate for higher levels of care, including inpatient treatment.

These guidelines are useful for making decisions related to level of care. They may not give an exact placement level for each patient, but they can simplify the process of making placement decisions.

CONCLUSION

Determining the appropriate level of care is a foundational component of eating disorder treatment and requires careful consideration of multiple factors. Medical and psychiatric stability, symptom severity, treatment history, motivation, and environmental supports must all be assessed to ensure that patients receive the care they need in the most suitable setting. Although guidelines from sources such as the American Psychiatric Association (2023) and Massachusetts General Hospital (Guarda & Schreyer, 2010) provide a strong foundation for decision-making, clinicians must also apply their professional judgment and consider the unique needs of each patient.

The evidence base supports the use of structured guidelines and level-of-care criteria to improve treatment outcomes and reduce the risk of relapse or hospitalization (Simpson et al., 2021; Anderson et al., 2017). While some individuals may do well in outpatient or intensive outpatient programs, others may require more intensive settings such as partial hospitalization, residential treatment, or inpatient hospitalization to address serious medical complications or co-occurring psychiatric conditions (Frostad & Bentz, 2022; Ulfvebrand et al., 2015). Recognizing that these decisions are nuanced and dependent on the patient's unique needs reinforces the importance of interdisciplinary collaboration and ongoing reassessment throughout the course of treatment. Ultimately, placing patients in an appropriate level-of-care increases the likelihood of recovery by matching them with the intensity of services required to meet their clinical needs.

REFERENCES

American Psychiatric Association. (2023). *Practice guideline for the treatment of patients with eating disorders* (4th ed.)., DOI: 10.1176/appi.books.9780890425862

Anderson, L. K., Reilly, E. E., Berner, L., Wierenga, C. E., Jones, M. D., Brown, T. A., Kaye, W. H., & Cusack, A. (2017). Treating eating disorders at higher levels of care: Overview and challenges. *Current Psychiatry Reports*, *19*(48), 48. Advance online publication. DOI: 10.1007/s11920-017-0796-4 PMID: 28653117

Bendall, C., & Taylor, N. F. (2023). The effect of oral refeeding compared with nasogastric refeeding on the quality of care for patients hospitalised with an eating disorder: A systematic review. *Nutrition & Dietetics: the Journal of the Dietitians Association of Australia*, *80*(1), 44–54. DOI: 10.1111/1747-0080.12770 PMID: 36254572

Frostad, S., & Bentz, M. (2022). Anorexia nervosa: Outpatient treatment and medical management. *World Journal of Psychiatry*, *12*(4), 558–579. DOI: 10.5498/wjp.v12.i4.558 PMID: 35582333

Graves, L. (n.d). *Levels of care.* National Eating Disorders Association. Retrieved June 13, 2025, from https://www.nationaleatingdisorders.org/levels-of-care/

Guarda, A. S., & Schreyer, C. C. (2010). Levels of care for eating disorders. In Herzog, D. B., Walsh, D. E., & Eddy, K. A. (Eds.), *Medical complications of eating disorders: A guide for professionals* (pp. 97–110). Massachusetts General Hospital and McGraw-Hill Medical.

Peckmezian, T., & Paxton, S. J. (2020). A systematic review of outcomes following residential treatment for eating disorders. *European Eating Disorders Review*, *28*(3), 246–259. DOI: 10.1002/erv.2733 PMID: 32196843

Simpson, C. C., Towne, T. L., Karam, A. M., Donahue, J. M., Hadjeasgari, C. F., Rockwell, R., & Kaye, W. H. (2021). Predictors of stepping up to higher level of care among eating disorder patients in a partial hospitalization program. *Frontiers in Psychology*, *12*, 667868. Advance online publication. DOI: 10.3389/fpsyg.2021.667868 PMID: 34366985

Ulfvebrand, S., Birgegård, A., Norring, C., Högdahl, L., & von Hausswolff-Juhlin, Y. (2015). Psychiatric comorbidity in women and men with eating disorders: Results from a large clinical database. *Psychiatry Research*, *230*(2), 294–299. DOI: 10.1016/j.psychres.2015.09.008 PMID: 26416590

KEY TERMS AND DEFINITIONS

Inpatient Hospitalization: A level of eating disorder treatment that occurs in a medical hospital to meet the immediate needs of patients who are medically unstable

Intensive Outpatient Programming: Eating disorder treatment that occurs in a community setting offering a range of services, with treatment occurring 3-5 days per week for around 3 hours per day

Medical Instability: A feature, evidenced by organ malfunction, low blood pressure or heart rate, low blood glucose, electrolyte imbalances, dehydration, or type 1 diabetes, requiring inpatient hospitalization in adults

Partial Hospitalization Program (PHP): An eating disorder treatment program that offers day treatment for 6-10 hours per day, up to 7 days a week

Residential Treatment: The level of eating disorder care that occurs in a home-like facility, where patients stay overnight and receive a variety of services; does not offer tube feeding

Standard Outpatient Treatment: The lowest level of care, typically characterized by attending psychotherapy once or twice weekly

Chapter 12
The Eating Disorder Treatment Team

ABSTRACT

This chapter discusses in detail the professionals who play a role in eating disorder treatment. It discusses the multidisciplinary approach that is the best practice in eating disorder care. The chapter also describes the roles of the various professionals involved in eating disorder treatment, including psychiatrists, dieticians, psychiatric nurses, psychologists, social workers, medical doctors, and professional counselors. The chapter concludes with an example of a multidisciplinary team in action.

INTRODUCTION

Earlier chapters in this text have discussed psychotherapy methods used in the treatment of eating disorders. Behavioral health professionals, including mental health counselors, clinical social workers, and psychologists typically provide psychotherapy. However, the reality is that one profession alone does not dominate the world of eating disorder treatment. Instead, treatment involves a multidisciplinary approach, with professionals collaborating to provide physical, psychological, psychiatric, and nutritional interventions (Monteleone et al., 2019). The American Psychiatric Association (2023) recommends that a multidisciplinary team provide services to ensure the best outcomes for patients. The sections that follow describe the key members of the eating disorder treatment

DOI: 10.4018/979-8-3373-0664-3.ch012

team, as well as the role that they play in patient recovery. While some professionals discussed in this chapter may provide the psychotherapeutic treatments detailed earlier, others provide complementary interventions that are essential for recovery.

KEY MULTIDISCIPLINARY TEAM MEMBERS

Best practices dictate that eating disorder treatment should occur via the coordinated efforts of a multidisciplinary team that has the expertise to provide psychological, psychiatric, nutritional, and medical treatment (American Psychiatric Association, 2023; Monteleone et al., 2019). As such, multiple different professions can play a critical role in the provision of evidence-based eating disorder treatment.

Psychiatrists

Psychiatrists are medical doctors who specialize in the treatment of mental health disorders; they can prescribe medication, in addition to providing talk therapy services. They are often viewed as the leaders of eating disorder treatment teams, as they can provide initial assessment, prescribe medication if warranted, and refer patients to other services, such as an inpatient hospitalization and mental health services (Monteleone et al., 2019). Psychiatrists in eating disorder treatment can provide comprehensive psychiatric assessments, prescribe medication, and manage any medications a patient is taking (Graves, n.d.). They may play a lead role in conducting a diagnostic assessment, and they must be prepared to conduct a full medical history to determine what medications are safe for the patient to take (Weltzin & Fitzpatrick, 2015).

Licensed Professional Counselors

Licensed professional counselors are masters-level trained clinicians who can provide a range of psychotherapy services. While psychiatrists are trained in psychotherapy methods, it is more likely that psychiatrists are providing medication management, while other professionals, including licensed professional counselors, offer talk therapy services. Depending on the jurisdiction in which one is practicing, some licensed professional counselors may be called licensed mental health counselors instead.

Psychologists

Psychologists are doctoral-level mental health professionals who are qualified to diagnose eating disorders and provide psychotherapy services. When providing therapy services, psychologists aim to identify the underlying problem contributing to the eating disorder and develop a treatment plan aimed at correcting problematic thoughts and behaviors linked to the disorder (American Psychological Association, 2020; Graves, n.d.).

Social Workers

Social workers can also be a part of the treatment team for eating disorders. Masters-level clinical social workers can provide therapy services (Graves, n.d.). Clinical social workers can evaluate client problems, including eating disorders, develop treatment plans, and help clients to change thoughts and behaviors. Clinical social workers, like psychologists, can diagnose mental illness and provide therapeutic modalities, such as family therapy, cognitive behavioral therapy, and group therapy (National Association of Social Workers, 2025). Social workers may also work in hospital settings and provide counseling services, as well as discharge planning and linkage to other resources.

Therapists

The term "therapist" is an umbrella term referring to a variety of different professions. Professional counselors, social workers, psychologists, and licensed mental health counselors may all refer to their role as being that of a therapist. All of these aforementioned professions can provide psychotherapy services, which involves using specific methods such as cognitive behavioral therapy to assist clients with overcoming personal problems and coping with mental illness in the context of a supportive helping relationship (Graves, n.d., National Association of Social Workers, 2025). What is most important to understand is that therapists play a central role in eating disorder treatment, and there are a number of professions that may fall under this umbrella. Therapists may not always take the lead role in eating disorder treatment, but they are an essential part of the multidisciplinary team, as psychological treatment is typically the first choice for treatment of eating disorders in both children and adults (Monteleone et al., 2022).

Medical Doctors

Medical doctors practicing general medicine or pediatrics are often part of the treatment team. Because individuals with eating disorders must be evaluated to determine their level of medical stability, medical doctors play a critical part in patient care. These professionals are likely to conduct medical histories, order and evaluate lab work, and determine if a patient requires medical treatment. In inpatient hospital settings, medical doctors may oversee services such a tube feeding or monitoring of organ functioning (American Psychiatric Association, 2023; Anderson et al., 2017).

Psychiatric Nurses

Across treatment settings, psychiatric nurses are typically part of patient care for eating disorders. Nurses can monitor compliance with treatment, evaluate medication side effects, detect medical problems, measure weight and vital signs, and provide frequent assessment and observation of patients (Weltzin & Fitzpatrick, 2015).

Dieticians

In eating disorder treatment, the dietician provides nutritional management to help the patient achieve normalization of eating patterns. Dieticians assess nutritional status, provide meal plans, and track patient progress (Weltzin & Fitzpatrick, 2015). Dieticians practicing in the area of eating disorder treatment must be prepared to tailor their interventions to the patient's unique needs. The ultimate goal of intervention by a dietician is to provide medical stabilization and to help patients meet nutritional requirements for recovery (Heafala et al., 2021).

Dieticians may also be responsible for providing education on the topic of nutrition, which includes discussion of metabolism, weight changes, typical eating patterns, myths related to food, and consequences of dieting and disordered eating. While patient education is a key role of dieticians in eating disorder treatment, these professionals may also educate other members of the treatment team on topics related to nutrition (Heafala et al., 2021).

THE EVIDENCE BASE SURROUNDING THE MULTIDISCIPLINARY APPROACH

A multidisciplinary team approach to eating disorder treatment is a recommended best practice (Bray et al., 2024). The effectiveness of multidisciplinary treatment models has been documented across care settings. For instance, Monteleone et al. (2019) argue that a multidisciplinary framework is essential for adapting treatment to individual differences in symptom severity, cultural background, and co-occurring conditions. Moreover, coordinated team-based care facilitates continuity of treatment as patients transition between levels of care, reducing the likelihood of relapse and improving long-term outcomes. A collaborative approach is considered best practice for all levels of care and has been shown to improve treatment adherence, symptom reduction, and patient satisfaction (Weltzin & Fitzpatrick, 2015).

Further evidence for the benefits of collaborative care models comes from studies focused on patient perspectives. Bray et al. (2024) found that individuals with lived experience of participating in outpatient treatment found value in the consistent communication among team members, shared treatment goals, and feeling heard and supported across disciplines. These themes were linked with higher satisfaction, reduced ambivalence about treatment, and increased motivation for recovery.

A growing body of research also highlights the potential for multidisciplinary care to alleviate fragmentation in the treatment system and reduce the burden on any single provider. For example, the National Eating Disorders Collaboration (NEDC, 2022) in Australia recommends integrated, team-based models of care as a way to improve accessibility and continuity of care for patients across community and inpatient settings. Their guidelines emphasize that coordinated treatment leads to better outcomes in weight restoration, psychological symptom reduction, and prevention of treatment dropout.

Finally, collaborative care allows for early identification and response to medical and psychological deterioration. Regular interdisciplinary meetings allow team members to identify emerging risks or challenges, including refeeding syndrome, suicidal ideation, or renewed purging behaviors, and adjust treatment plans proactively. This level of monitoring and flexibility enhances clinical safety and responsiveness, particularly in higher levels of care such as partial hospitalization or residential treatment (Anderson et al., 2017).

Given the complex nature of eating disorders, a siloed approach to care is inadequate. Instead, treatment teams must communicate regularly, share observations, and revise treatment plans collaboratively to ensure a unified and person-centered approach. This model is endorsed by both national and international clinical guidelines and should be considered a standard of care at all levels of treatment.

The Multidisciplinary Approach in Action

It can be helpful to review an example of the multidisciplinary eating disorder team in action. Consider a patient, Marcella, who is entering a residential treatment program for bulimia nervosa. She was initially seen by her family medicine doctor, who reviewed her medical history and current symptoms. Marcella's family doctor identified that she had a history of bulimia nervosa alongside bipolar disorder. Marcella revealed that she has no control over her binging and purging episodes, which are occurring multiple times per day. Fortunately, Marcella's family doctor finds that Marcella has no pressing medical concerns, but given Marcella's symptom severity and the presence of co-occurring bipolar disorder, the family doctor and Marcella agree that residential treatment is the best setting for Marcella's care. Once Marcella arrives at the residential facility, she meets with a psychiatrist, who performs a full diagnostic assessment, reviews Marcella's medical history, and evaluates the need for medication. She also sees a psychiatric nurse, who measures vital signs and documents Marcella's weight upon arrival. Marcella is ultimately prescribed a mood stabilizer to manage symptoms of bipolar disorder.

After arriving at the facility, Marcella meets her primary therapist and her nutritionist. Based on the psychiatrist's diagnosis and assessment, the therapist, who is a licensed professional counselor, determines that psychodynamic therapy aimed at meeting unmet attachment needs is the best approach for Marcella. Marcella's nutritionist evaluates Marcella's eating patterns and provides her with psychoeducation related to the role that restriction plays in promoting binge-eating. The nutritionist also helps Marcella to normalize her eating habits by eating three snacks and two nutritious meals per day. In addition to receiving services from her therapist and nutritionist, Marcella also regularly checks in with nurses to monitor her weight and medication side effects. Marcella shares with other patients during group settings led by a licensed social worker, and these sessions are helpful for connecting Marcella with social support.

As Marcella progresses through treatment, her multidisciplinary team meets regularly to discuss her progress. The nurse notes that Marcella is responding well to her medication with no significant side effects. At one point, the therapist reports that Marcella discloses continued urges to binge-eat, which prompts the nutritionist to check in and ensure that Marcella is not restricting. A nurse is assigned to monitor Marcella more closely during mealtimes to ensure she is not restricting food intake. Over time, Marcella is able to normalize her eating patterns and reduce urges to binge-eat and purge. During a team meeting, the psychiatrist, who leads Marcella's treatment team, suggests that Marcella is ready for discharge, and other team members agree. In consultation with the other team members, the psychiatrist develops a discharge plan, which includes referral to an intensive outpatient program offering individual therapy, group therapy, and nutritional counseling so that Marcella can continue with her treatment.

As demonstrated in the example above, a multidisciplinary team ensures that a patient receives comprehensive treatment, with all of their treatment needs met. As shown in the example, the psychiatrist leads the team and ensures that a patient receives needed medication, while the nurse can provide regular monitoring. The therapist offers psychological services to address underlying issues contributing to disordered eating, while the nutritionist helps the patient to normalize eating habits. Regular communication among team members allows adjustments to be made, as needed. For instance, if the therapist provides feedback that the patient has urges to binge-eat, the nutritionist, in turn, may need to make adjustments, which the nurse can support. Ultimately, the team can provide better care to the patient than any single team member could on their own.

CONCLUSION

The effective treatment of eating disorders requires the expertise and coordinated efforts of a multidisciplinary team. No single provider can address the full spectrum of medical, psychological, and nutritional complexities associated with these conditions. When each team member—whether psychiatrist, psychologist, dietitian, social worker, nurse, or physician—contributes their specialized knowledge within a collaborative team, patient care is more complete and more effective. Research has consistently shown that multidisciplinary teams improve treatment engagement, reduce relapse risk, and support long-term recovery (Bray et al., 2024; Monteleone et al., 2019; Weltzin & Fitzpatrick, 2015). By integrating diverse perspectives and sharing treatment goals, these teams provide patient-centered care that adapts to evolving needs and promotes continuity across levels of care. As the field advances, fostering strong multidisciplinary collaboration must remain a central priority in the design and delivery of effective eating disorder services.

REFERENCES

American Psychiatric Association. (2023). *Practice guideline for the treatment of patients with eating disorders* (4th ed.)., DOI: 10.1176/appi.books.9780890425862

American Psychological Association. (2020, February 25). *Eating disorders: How psychotherapy can help people recover.* https://www.apa.org/topics/eating-disorders/psychotherapy

Anderson, L. K., Reilly, E. E., Berner, L., Wierenga, C. E., Jones, M. D., Brown, T. A., Kaye, W. H., & Cusack, A. (2017). Treating eating disorders at higher levels of care: Overview and challenges. *Current Psychiatry Reports*, *19*(48), 48. Advance online publication. DOI: 10.1007/s11920-017-0796-4 PMID: 28653117

Bray, M., Heruc, G., Evans, L., & Wright, O. R. L. (2024). The imperative of collaboration: Lived experience perspectives on team approaches in outpatient eating disorder treatment. *International Journal of Eating Disorders*, *57*(1), 116–123. DOI: 10.1002/eat.24084 PMID: 37902406

Graves, L. (n.d). *Levels of care.* National Eating Disorders Association. Retrieved June 13, 2025, from https://www.nationaleatingdisorders.org/levels-of-care/

Heafala, A., Ball, L., Rayner, J., & Mitchell, L. J. (2021). What role do dietitians have in providing nutrition care for eating disorder treatment? An integrative review. *Journal of Human Nutrition and Dietetics*, *34*(4), 724–735. DOI: 10.1111/jhn.12927 PMID: 34031923

Monteleone, A., Pellegrino, F., Croatto, G., Carfagno, M., Hilbert, A., Treasure, J., Wade, T., Bulik, C. M., Zipfel, S., Hay, P., Schmidt, U., Castellini, G., Favaro, A., Fernandez-Aranda, F., Il Shin, J., Voderholzer, U., Ricca, V., Moretti, D., Busatta, D., & Solmi, M. (2022). Treatment of eating disorders: A systematic meta-review of meta- analyses and network meta-analyses. *Neuroscience and Biobehavioral Reviews*, *142*, 104857. DOI: 10.1016/j.neubiorev.2022.104857 PMID: 36084848

Monteleone, A. M., Fernandez-Aranda, F., & Voderholzer, U. (2019). Evidence and perspectives in eating disorders: A paradigm for a multidisciplinary approach. *World Psychiatry; Official Journal of the World Psychiatric Association (WPA)*, *18*(3), 369–370. DOI: 10.1002/wps.20687 PMID: 31496108

National Association of Social Workers. (2025). *NASW standards for clinical social work in social work practice* (©2025). NASW Press. https://www.socialworkers.org/Practice/NASW-Practice-Standards-Guidelines/NASW-Standards-for-Clinical-Social-Work-in-Social-Work-Practice

National Eating Disorders Collaboration. (2022). *Eating disorders: A professional resource for general practitioners*. https://www.nedc.com.au/assets/NEDC-Resources/NEDC- Resource-GPs.pdf

Weltzin, T. E., & Fitzpatrick, M. E. (2015). The eating disorders treatment team and continuum of care. In Smolak, L., & Levine, M. P. (Eds.), *The Wiley handbook of eating disorders*. Wiley., DOI: 10.1002/9781118574089.ch50

KEY TERMS AND DEFINITIONS

Dietician: A member of the eating disorder treatment team who helps patients to normalize eating patterns, learn about nutrition topics, and develop meal plans

Medical doctor: A general physician who determines a patient's level of medical stability and provides medical treatments, including in the inpatient hospital setting

Professional Counselor: A mental health provider who can provide therapy services; may also be titled a mental health counselor

Psychiatric Nurse: A member of the eating disorder treatment team who provides observation and assessment and supports the work of medical doctors and psychiatrists

Psychiatrist: A medical doctor specifically trained to diagnose and treat mental illnesses, primarily through the use of medications

Psychologist: A doctoral-level mental health professional who can diagnose and treat mental health disorders

Psychotherapy: A service that involves treatment of mental health disorders through the use of clinical services aimed at helping clients improve coping and problem-solving in the context of a supportive relationship

Social Worker: An eating disorder treatment team member who can provide therapy services and also assist with discharge planning

Therapist: An umbrella term used to describe mental health professionals who offer psychotherapy services

Chapter 13
Cultural Considerations in Eating Disorder Treatment

ABSTRACT

This chapter addresses concepts related to cultural diversity, cultural sensitivity, and cultural competence in eating disorder treatment. It begins with a discussion of cultural norms related to eating and body image, including the fact that these norms are social constructs that vary by culture. The chapter further addresses how treatment may need to be modified to meet the needs of diverse cultural groups. Finally, the chapter concludes with a discussion of the ethics of culturally competent care and specific strategies for addressing cultural needs in eating disorder treatment.

INTRODUCTION

Eating disorders are complex mental health conditions that occur across diverse cultural groups. However, most research and treatment models have historically focused on white, Western, cisgender female populations. In fact, a recent review of 377 research manuscripts found that in studies that reported data on race and ethnicity, White participants made up around 70% of samples (Egbert et al., 2022). This narrow scope has led to underdiagnosis, misdiagnosis, and inadequate care for individuals from racially, ethnically, and culturally diverse backgrounds (Acle et al.,

DOI: 10.4018/979-8-3373-0664-3.ch013

2021). Integrating cultural considerations into eating disorder treatment is essential to ensure equitable care and improve treatment outcomes across populations; researchers must also be committed to evaluating the effectiveness of assessment tools and interventions with groups historically underrepresented in research. That being said, it is essential to consider a patient's cultural needs when selecting an evidence-based treatment modality. This chapter discusses cultural needs in detail, to ensure that practitioners are prepared to provide culturally-informed services.

CULTURAL INFLUENCES ON THE DEVELOPMENT AND EXPRESSION OF EATING DISORDERS

Culture plays a significant role in shaping body image ideals, eating behaviors, and the meanings people ascribe to food and weight. In eating disorder treatment, the concept of body image, which refers to the emotions and perceptions one has related to their body, as well as how satisfied or dissatisfied they are with their body, plays a central role. Because perceptions of the ideal body are socially constructed, culture contributes significantly to body image, and thus eating disorder treatment. Thinness tends to be idealized in Western cultures, including in the United States, Canada, and England. In Asian countries, including China and Japan, the preference for a slim build can lead to body image disturbances and eating disorders, especially in adolescent girls. Alternatively, African culture tends to accept greater diversity in body types. While urban areas may follow Western standards related to thinness as the ideal, rural African communities are less likely to be influenced by the thin ideal, which views slimmer bodies as superior. In Latin America, body dissatisfaction is common, but the Western thin ideal doesn't exert as much of an influence. Finally, women may be subjected to different body standards based upon what is attractive to the opposite sex within their cultural group. For example, African American men have been found to prefer women in larger bodies when compared to White men (Abdoli et al., 2024).

Internalization of the thin ideal can be particularly concerning from the standpoint of eating disorder experts, because it is linked to both eating and weight concerns. The relationship between the thin ideal and eating and weight concerns appears to be consistent across ethnic groups. However, African Americans score lower than all other ethnic identified groups on internalization of the thin ideal (Rakhkovskaya & Warren, 2014).

The cultural differences noted above can cause individuals with disordered eating behaviors to present differently, based on their cultural context. For instance, when compared to White women, African American women living with binge-eating disorder may be less likely to be concerned about binge-eating, weight, and body shape. Similarly, Asian American women with anorexia nervosa may not demonstrate fear of becoming overweight, which is one of the diagnostic criteria for the disorder. Based on differences in presentation, some individuals with disordered eating behaviors may not meet the diagnostic threshold for a specific disorder, and thus may be seen as not requiring treatment, when, in fact, they are in need of support (Acle et al., 2021).

Furthermore, acculturation challenges and identity conflict can contribute to disordered eating. Acculturation can be described as cultural and psychological change that occurs when a person of one cultural group comes into contact with another cultural group. Research suggests that the acculturation process may make people more vulnerable to eating disorders. For instance, someone coming to the United States from a non-Western culture will be exposed to cultural ideals that dictate that thinness is superior to other body types. This can lead to disordered eating in an attempt to assimilate into the dominant culture. Integration, in which a person maintains their original cultural identity but also adopts the new cultural values, may be protective against disordered eating behaviors. Nonetheless, the process of adapting to a new culture can cause social and psychological distress, called acculturative stress, which occurs in response to the challenges linked to cultural change. The research suggests that cultural change and acculturative stress are linked to bulimic symptoms, binge-eating, and restrictive eating (Song et al. 2023).

TREATMENT BARRIERS IN CULTURALLY DIVERSE POPULATIONS

Beyond cultural variations in the expression of eating disorder symptoms and norms related to the ideal body, some cultural groups may lack access to quality eating disorder treatment. Many people from racially and ethnically marginalized groups face barriers to accessing and receiving effective treatment for eating disorders (Moreno et al. 2023). Barriers include stigma, lack of culturally competent providers, language barriers, and financial constraints (Acle et al., 2021; Goel et al., 2023). Additionally, health care professionals may hold implicit biases or stereotypes that interfere with accurate assessment and referral (Acle et al., 2021). For instance, research has found that clinicians are less likely to detect eating disorders in African American girls when compared to Caucasian or Hispanic girls, indicating that professionals may act according to race-based stereotypes and therefore fail to diagnose eating disorders in African American girls (Gordon et al., 2006). Some research has found that clinicians are less likely to detect eating disorders in Hispanic girls as well. This may occur because of the misconception that only Caucasian girls are vulnerable to eating disorders, since their cultural values support thinness as the ideal. However, the reality is that African American and Hispanic girls are exposed to dominant culture ideals, and they may be more influenced by these norms than the norms of their own cultures (Gordon et al., 2002). When a clinician operates according to a racial stereotype and fails to detect an eating disorder, patients may go without needed treatment.

Individuals belonging to racial or ethnic minority groups are not the only population that may experience barriers to effective eating disorder treatment. For example, members of the LGBTQ+ population may feel isolated and misunderstood in treatment settings, which could prevent them from experiencing the full benefits of treatment. Individuals who are part of the LGBTQ+ community may feel as if treatment is not designed for them, since it is likely to be based on heteronormative structures. Patients who identify as transgender are particularly at-risk of poor experiences in eating disorder treatment, especially if providers do not understand the link between gender dysphoria and eating disorders (White et al., 2024). Lack of treatment that supports the needs of LGBTQ+ communities is a serious injustice, as sexual and gender minority populations are more likely to experience anorexia nervosa, bulimia nervosa, and binge-eating disorder during their lifetimes when compared to cisgender, heterosexual populations. Minority stress and discrimination can fuel body dissatisfaction and disordered eating (Nagata et al., 2020), making LGBT+ populations particularly vulnerable to eating disorders.

CULTURAL ADAPTATIONS IN EATING DISORDER TREATMENT

Because culture can influence body image ideals and eating disorder symptom presentation, evidence-based treatments may require adaptation to meet the needs of culturally diverse groups. When providing interventions to patients from cultures that do not follow Western ideals, clinicians may also have to adjust their communication style and recommendations to meet cultural needs. For instance, cognitive behavioral therapy (CBT) has been identified as beneficial for treating bulimia nervosa; however, Japanese women may not respond as positively to the standard form of CBT, based on their cultural needs. They may view the suggested behavioral changes as being aggressive. Furthermore, based on the standard Japanese diet of rice and fermented foods, the normalization of eating habits may look different in Japanese compared to Western populations. So, when providing CBT to Japanese populations, the clinician will likely need to adapt the modality to use gentler, less directive language and to include foods from Japanese culture when providing psychoeducation on the normalization of eating habits (Hamatani et al., 2022).

Research with Latina populations has demonstrated that cognitive behavioral therapy for bulimia nervosa (CBT-BN) is generally effective for this population, and clinicians do not need to make any major adaptations to core CBT-BN interventions. However, Latina patients are likely to be more engaged in treatment when the clinician integrates their cultural values into sessions. For instance, Latina culture tends to emphasize familism, a cultural norm that values family support, family loyalty, and family obligations. To integrate these values into treatment sessions, clinicians can include spouses in the treatment process or include family-related goals, such as improved parenting skills, in the treatment plan. Finally, Latina patients may prefer a clinician of the same ethnicity to help them feel understood (Reyes-Rodriguez et al., 2014).

Additionally, Black Americans may have different treatment needs when compared to those of the dominant culture. For instance, when treating binge-eating disorder, Blacks may not identify with weight loss as a treatment goal, so it's essential for clinicians to be mindful of this preference (Acle et al., 2021). Furthermore, experiences of oppression, including racism, classism, and sizeism, can contribute to disempowerment and anxiety in Black, Indigenous, and People of Color (BIPOC) populations. Clinicians must consider this when engaging with these populations. Research suggests that mindfulness-based approaches can be particularly helpful for assisting BIPOC patients with overcoming the anxiety associated with acculturative stress. Through mindfulness exercises, patients can learn to accept and experience emotions, rather than coping through disordered eating (Emelianchik-Key et al., 2023).

Finally, clinicians must consider the cultural needs of individuals who belong to the LGBTQ+ community. Individuals who belong to this community require compassionate care in safe spaces that affirm their identities. LGBTQ+ populations must feel as if they are accepted by treatment providers, otherwise they may hide their identities, which can impede treatment progress, since identity and eating disorder symptoms are inextricably intertwined. Compassionate care that is gender-affirming and trauma-informed can increase the effectiveness of eating disorder treatment in LGBTQ+ populations and strengthen the therapeutic alliance (White et al., 2024).

THE ETHICS OF CULTURAL COMPETENCE

Work aimed at promoting cultural competence in eating disorder treatment not only improves treatment outcomes for minoritized populations; it's also ethically required. For instance, the Code of Ethics of the National Association of Social Workers (NASW) calls upon social workers to address social injustices, which requires a commitment to understanding the influences of oppression and demonstrating sensitivity toward cultural diversity. Furthermore, social workers are ethically obligated to provide culturally competent services that empower marginalized groups (NASW, 2021). Social workers play a central role in providing therapy services to patients with eating disorders; therefore, they must be prepared to work with clients from different cultural backgrounds, showing sensitivity to cultural differences and experiences of oppression, which may impact service provision.

The American Psychological Association's (APA) Ethical Principles of Psychologists and Code of Conduct also calls upon psychologists to be sensitive to cultural diversity, albeit less explicitly than the NASW Code of Ethics. The APA Code of Conduct includes the general principle of justice, which emphasizes that all people must be able to access effective psychological services and that psychologists must ensure that biases do not contribute to unjust practices (APA, 2017). Given the APA's ethical position, psychologists in eating disorder treatment must also become culturally competent, so they can provide supportive, unbiased services that meet the needs of diverse cultural groups.

Other members of the eating disorder treatment team are also bound to ethical codes that address cultural competence. The Code of Ethics for Nurses from the American Nurses Association (2015) promotes the concept of allyship, which calls upon nurses to advocate for the elimination of harmful treatment and to ensure that there is space for all voices in the healthcare setting. Furthermore, nurses are ethically required to recognize the negative effects of oppression, bias, and discrimination on patient care and to provide culturally-appropriate services (American Nurses Association, 2015). Based on these standards in the ethics code, nurses working in eating disorder treatment must also be prepared to provide culturally-sensitive services. Finally, the Code of Ethics for the Nutrition and Dietetics Profession (2018), highlights the importance of being mindful of difference and diversity.

ENSURING CULTURALLY-SENSITIVE PRACTICES

Given the importance of cultural competence and consideration of cultural differences in eating disorder treatment, professionals must be prepared to actively promote cultural sensitivity in practice. This means having an understanding of patients' cultural needs and providing treatments that consider a patient's experiences of marginalization, as well as the cultural values that might inform evidence-based treatment. Cultural sensitivity begins during the assessment process. Cultural formulation tools, such as the Cultural Formulation Interview (CFI) from DSM-5-TR, provide a structured method for assessing the impact of culture on an individual's experience and treatment preferences (American Psychiatric Association, 2022). Involving family and community members who understand the patient's cultural background can also enhance engagement and support recovery (Reyes-Rodriguez et al., 2014).

Additionally, clinician training is essential for promoting culturally-competent practice. Providers should be trained to recognize and address their own implicit biases and to adapt their clinical approach to respect the individual's cultural framework. This includes being aware of how privilege, oppression, and systemic inequities may intersect with the eating disorder experience (NASW, 2021). Training in work with specific populations, such as the LBGTQ+ community, is warranted, especially among clinicians working in settings serving significant numbers of individuals from this population (White et al., 2024).

It is beyond the scope of this textbook to provide specific guidance related to the cultural needs of every patient a clinician may encounter in practice. However, the following guidelines, based on the findings of a recent systematic review, provide general strategies that eating disorder treatment professionals may use to promote culturally competent care (Acle et al., 2021):

- Consider working with alternative medicine providers or community leaders, should the patient come from a non-Western culture or express preference for inclusion of these members in the treatment plan.
- Be mindful of and prepared to address barriers to treatment-seeking, such as stigma, shame, and financial limitations.
- Conduct an assessment of the patient's cultural context, which includes exploring the meanings they assign to weight, body image, and diet, as well as the norms related to these concepts.

- Assess factors including gender, cultural values, social class, ableism, and educational attainment as well as any trauma related to these factors.
- Operate from a posture of curiosity and non-judgment toward clients, which creates safety, makes clients the experts of their lived experiences, and promotes a strong therapeutic alliance.
- Recognize that cultural variations in symptom presentation can result in some patients demonstrating subthreshold symptoms or experiencing body image concerns related to facial features, for instance, rather than body weight.
- Evaluate family and social supports and be prepared to provide psychoeducation about eating disorders.
- Assess a patient's level of acculturation and acculturative stress.
- Seek education and training on the topic of working with racial and ethnic minorities and commit to acknowledging diversity while avoiding the perpetuation of stereotypes.

CONCLUSION

Cultural considerations are not optional but essential in the treatment of eating disorders. By acknowledging and incorporating cultural factors into assessment, diagnosis, and treatment, clinicians can improve engagement, reduce disparities, and enhance outcomes for individuals from all backgrounds. A culturally responsive framework is necessary for ethically sound and effective eating disorder care. Clinicians who feel they are lacking cultural competence should seek training, especially when working with diverse populations. It's also important for clinicians to remember that a commitment to cultural competence requires ongoing learning.

REFERENCES

Abdoli, M., Rosato, M. S., Desousa, A., & Cotrufo, P. (2024). Cultural differences in body image: A systematic review. *Social Sciences (Basel, Switzerland), 13*(6), 305. DOI: 10.3390/socsci13060305

Acle, A., Cook, B. J., & Beasley, T. (2021). Cultural considerations in the treatment of eating disorders among racial/ethnic minorities: A systematic review. *Journal of Cross-Cultural Psychology*, *52*(5), 379–399. DOI: 10.1177/00220221211017664

American Nurses Association. (2015). *Code of ethics for nurses with interpretive statements* (2nd ed.). American Nurses Publishing.

American Psychiatric Association. (2022). Diagnostic and statistical manual of mental disorders (5th ed., text rev.)., , DSM-5-TR.DOI: 10.1176/appi.books.9780890425787

American Psychological Association. (2017). *Ethical principles of psychologists and code of conduct* (2002, Amended June 1, 2010, and January 1, 2017). https://www.apa.org/ethics/code

Egbert, A. H., Hunt, R. A., Williams, K. L., Burke, N. L., & Mathis, K. J. (2022). Reporting racial and ethnic diversity in eating disorder research over the past 20 years. *International Journal of Eating Disorders*, *55*(4), 455–462. DOI: 10.1002/eat.23666 PMID: 34997609

Emelianchik-Key, K., Labarta, A., & Gill, C. S. (2023). The mediating role of transdiagnostic factors in a clinical sample of Black, Indigenous, and People of Color with eating disorders. *Journal of Mental Health Counseling*, *45*(4), 340–356. DOI: 10.17744/mehc.45.4.04

Goel, N. J., Thomas, B., Boutté, R. L., Kaur, B., & Mazzeo, S. E. (2023). "What will people say?": Mental health stigmatization as a barrier to eating disorder treatment-seeking for South Asian American women. *Asian American Journal of Psychology*, *14*(1), 96–113. DOI: 10.1037/aap0000271 PMID: 37283957

Gordon, K. H., Brattole, M. M., Wingate, L. R., & Joiner, T. E.Jr. (2006). The impact of client race on clinician detection of eating disorders. *Behavior Therapy*, *37*(4), 319–325. DOI: 10.1016/j.beth.2005.12.002 PMID: 17071210

Gordon, K. H., Perez, M., & Joiner, T. E.Jr. (2002). The impact of racial stereotypes on eating disorder recognition. *International Journal of Eating Disorders*, *32*(2), 219–224. DOI: 10.1002/eat.10070 PMID: 12210665

Hamatani, S., Matsumoto, K., Ishibashi, T., Shibukawa, R., Honda, Y., Kosaka, H., Mizuno, Y., & Andersson, G. (2022). Development of a culturally adaptable internet-based cognitive behavioral therapy for Japanese women with bulimia nervosa. *Frontiers in Psychiatry*, *13*(942936), 942936. Advance online publication. DOI: 10.3389/fpsyt.2022.942936 PMID: 36081468

Moreno, R., Buckelew, S. M., Accurso, E. C., & Raymond-Flesch, M. (2023). Disparities in access to eating disorders treatment for publicly-insured youth and youth of color: A retrospective cohort study. *Journal of Eating Disorders*, *11*(10), 10. Advance online publication. DOI: 10.1186/s40337-022-00730-7 PMID: 36694235

Nagata, J. M., Ganson, K. T., & Austin, S. B. (2020). Emerging trends in eating disorders among sexual and gender minorities. *Current Opinion in Psychiatry*, *33*(6), 562–567. DOI: 10.1097/YCO.0000000000000645 PMID: 32858597

National Association of Social Workers. (2021). *Code of ethics of the National Association of Social Workers*. https://www.socialworkers.org/About/Ethics/Code-of-Ethics/Code-of-Ethics-English/Social-Workers-Ethical-Responsibilities-to-Clients

Rakhkovskaya, L. M., & Warren, C. S. (2014). Ethnic identity, thin-ideal internalization, and eating pathology in ethnically diverse college women. *Body Image*, *11*(4), 438–445. DOI: 10.1016/j.bodyim.2014.07.003 PMID: 25079012

Reyes-Rodriguez, M. L., Baucom, D. H., & Bulik, C. M. (2014). Culturally sensitive intervention for Latina women with eating disorders: A case study. *Revista Mexicana de Trastornos Alimentarios*, *5*(2), 136–146. DOI: 10.1016/S2007-1523(14)72009-9 PMID: 25598951

Song, S., Stern, C. M., Deitsch, T., & Sala, M. (2023). Acculturation and eating disorders: A systematic review. *Eating and Weight Disorders*, *28*(39), 39. Advance online publication. DOI: 10.1007/s40519-023-01563-2 PMID: 37076614

White, M., Thomas, A., Aston, M., & Joy, P. (2024). "It's beautiful and it's messy and it's tragic": Exploring the role of compassion in the eating disorder recovery processes of 2S/LGBTQ+ Canadians. *Journal of Eating Disorders*, *12*(23), 23. Advance online publication. DOI: 10.1186/s40337-024-00981-6 PMID: 38326869

KEY TERMS AND DEFINITIONS

Acculturation: The process of psychological and cultural change that occurs as a result of a person from one cultural group coming into contact with another cultural group

Acculturative Stress: A specific type of social and psychological distress resulting from the challenges associated with cultural change

Body Image: Perceptions and emotions related to the body, including one's level of satisfaction or dissatisfaction with their body

Familism: A cultural norm often seen in Latino cultures that views family support, family loyalty, and family obligations as paramount

Integration: A process by which a person coming into contact with a new culture retains pieces of their old culture while also adopting new cultural values

Justice: A general principle in the American Psychological Association's Ethical Principles of Psychologists and Code of Conduct that states all people must be able to access quality psychological services

Thin ideal: A standard in Western cultures that views slender bodies as being superior to larger bodies

Chapter 14
Gaps in Knowledge and Future Directions

ABSTRACT

This chapter discusses current gaps in knowledge with respect to evidence-based eating disorder treatment. The chapter addresses the fact that much research in the realm of evidence-based eating disorder treatments uses White, cisgender populations, which leads to disparities in treatment quality. It also evaluates gaps in areas such as treatment of severe and enduring anorexia nervosa and in evidence-based practices promoting sustained remission. Furthermore, the chapter includes a discussion of the gap between research and practice and concludes with a discussion of emerging treatments, including digital interventions and treatments based on the results of genetic and neurological studies.

INTRODUCTION

Despite decades of clinical advancement and increased awareness, eating disorder research and treatment continue to suffer from significant gaps. While evidence-based treatments such as cognitive-behavioral therapy (CBT), family-based therapy (FBT), and dialectical behavior therapy (DBT) have demonstrated efficacy (Ben-Porath et al., 2020; Brockmeyer et al., 2018) large segments of the population remain underserved or poorly understood (Acle et al., 2021; Penwell et al., 2024; Rodgers et al., 2018). There are also emerging treatment modalities that show promise

DOI: 10.4018/979-8-3373-0664-3.ch014

but require further evidence to support their use. This chapter critically evaluates gaps in knowledge and explores future directions for both treatment and research, grounded in current empirical findings.

UNDERREPRESENTED POPULATIONS IN RESEARCH AND TREATMENT

One of the most pressing gaps in the research on evidence-based eating disorder treatments is the underrepresentation of marginalized populations in eating disorder research, including racial and ethnic minorities, LGBTQ+ individuals, people in larger bodies, and those with lower socioeconomic status (SES). Historically, eating disorders have been mischaracterized as disorders primarily affecting affluent White women, which has skewed research samples and clinical training (Goel et al., 2022; Sonneville & Lipson, 2018). Unfortunately, marginalized populations may not receive needed treatment under the current system that fails to detect eating disorders in these populations and fails to ensure equitable treatment access. For instance, one recent study found disparities in treatment access among youth of color and youth covered by public health insurance programs. Compared to those with private health insurance, youth with public health insurance are only one-third as likely to receive treatment. Furthermore, study results revealed that Latinx and Asian youth were half as likely to receive needed treatment when compared to White youth (Moreno et al., 2023). Additionally, transgender, non-binary, and sexual minority populations report higher rates of disordered eating than heterosexual, cisgender populations, but often face stigma and isolation in clinical settings (Nagata el al., 2020; White et al., 2024).

With marginalized groups being underrepresented in research, they continue to have eating disorder symptoms that go undetected and undertreated. When these groups do access treatment, it may not be culturally-sensitive, since most of the existing research is based on White populations. To address this gap, the Eating Disorders Research Society has focused on a justice, equity, diversity, and inclusion (JEDI) model which seeks to ensure that diverse groups of participants are recruited for eating disorder research, which in turn ensures that study results generalize to underrepresented groups. This model calls upon leaders in the research field to recruit researchers from underrepresented backgrounds so that research questions and methods better represent the diversity of populations served. Researchers themselves must also commit to conducting studies that enhance the understanding of eating disorders in historically underserved groups, rather than utilizing homogenous samples of White women from Western cultures (Goel et al., 2022).

LIMITED TREATMENT OPTIONS FOR SEVERE AND ENDURING ANOREXIA (SE-AN)

The term severe and enduring anorexia (SE-AN) is applied to cases in which anorexia persists, sometimes in a life-long fashion, usually with several bouts of unsuccessful treatment. Researchers have come to define SE-AN as a disorder that lasts more than three years and does not improve with exposure to two evidence-based treatments. Unfortunately, there is a lack of established evidence-based treatments for SE-AN, which is concerning given the potentially fatal nature of the disorder (Wonderlich et al., 2020).

To establish evidence-based treatment for the SE-AN, researchers have recommended the potential inclusion of a subcategory for this presentation in the DSM-5. Research should emphasize how to engage patients with this presentation of anorexia nervosa in treatment, how to support parents and caretakers of individuals with this disorder, and how to adapt existing treatments to meet the needs of patients with SE-AN. Additional research may reveal new treatment approaches for SE-AN or explore the biology underlying persistent versus shorter duration cases of anorexia nervosa (Wonderlich et al., 2020).

LACK OF LONG-TERM REMISSION WITH TREATMENT

Although short-term treatment outcomes are frequently reported, long-term follow up data are less common. Many studies evaluate outcomes at discharge or within one year post-treatment, but this leaves questions about the possibility of sustained recovery unanswered. A recent review of over 10 years of research found that there is a lack of research involving long-term follow up. For anorexia nervosa, the current research base shows a high mortality risk and low rates of remission, even when evidence-based treatments are utilized (Miskovic-Wheatley et al., 2023).

While studies involving long-term follow-up are few in number, the limited research that is available shows that many people do not achieve sustained recovery after completing treatment. For instance, one study that followed patients for 17 years found that only 29% of people remained fully recovered, while half remained ill. Additionally, relapse rates are significantly high, with as many as 41% of people relapsing by the second year after treatment discharge. Based on what is known from the existing research, additional studies must be conducted, using long-term follow up to evaluate the proportion of patients relapsing versus achieving remission. It's also essential to evaluate which evidence-based treatments, if any, are effective for promoting sustained recovery (Miskovic-Wheatley et al., 2023).

THE RESEARCH-PRACTICE GAP

Researchers in psychology and psychiatry have also identified that there is a "research-practice gap" in the field of eating disorder treatment. This refers to the disconnection between what researchers know about effective treatment, and what sort of treatment patients actually receive. In one study, just 32.7% of patients received a treatment defined as minimally adequate based recommendations related to evidence-based interventions. Among clinicians who specialize in treating eating disorders, only 6%-35% actually provide evidence-based treatments according to established treatment manuals and protocols (Kazdin et al., 2017).

The research-practice gap may exist, at least in part, because of a lack of competence related to eating disorder treatment among mental health professionals. Smith (2023) determined that there is a lack of professionals trained in the provision of evidence-based eating disorder interventions. Furthermore, MacCaughelty (2023) found that over half of the clinical social workers in their study did not assess for eating disorders within a patient's first two therapy sessions, and a lack of education was a leading reason for neglecting to conduct such assessment. The results of a recent study suggested that the lack of competence related to eating disorder treatment begins during a clinician's university education, as university faculty members reported being largely unprepared to deliver curriculum related to eating disorder (Author, 2025). Ultimately, while there is a rather significant evidence base related to effective eating disorder treatments, a substantial number of clinicians are not utilizing these treatments. It seems they may not even be learning about these treatments during their time enrolled in a university program.

EMERGING TREATMENTS

While there are gaps in knowledge within the eating disorder treatment arena, there are emerging areas of inquiry that may expand the understanding of eating disorders in the future. For instance, research may increase our understanding of genetic contributions to eating disorders, paving the way for treatments that target biological vulnerabilities. Furthermore, the expansion of technology can open the door to new treatments, delivered to patients in remote settings. Some of the emerging treatments that currently have the attention of researchers are described below.

Insights Related to Genetics and Neuroscience

Advances in neuroscience and genetics may provide insights into potential treatments. Recently, genome-wide association studies (GWAS) have revealed specific genes linked to anorexia nervosa. One large study used data from nearly 17,000 people with anorexia nervosa and over 55,000 people without the disorder and identified eight specific areas of the genome linked to anorexia, including four specific genes: CADM1, MGMT, FOXP1, and PTBP2. These genes were mostly active in the brain, especially in areas related to memory, emotion, and decision-making, like the hippocampus, striatum, and prefrontal cortex. This supports the idea that anorexia nervosa is influenced by brain biology as well as psychological and social factors (Bulik et al., 2022).

GWAS have also revealed that individuals with anorexia nervosa tend to share some of the same genetic risk factors as people with obsessive-compulsive disorder. Interestingly, some of these shared genes are active in the prefrontal cortex, which plays a role in decision-making, self-control, and regulating emotions. This link may explain why both anorexia nervosa and obsessive-compulsive disorder involve rigid thinking patterns, obsessive thoughts, and repetitive behaviors, such as compulsive exercise or ritualistic behaviors (Bulik et al., 2022).

While studies in the field of genetics and neuroscience have limited clinical use currently, they may prove useful as additional research unfolds. Scientists aim to translate the findings of research into the development of biologically-informed treatments. This might involve the formulation of pharmacological treatments that address core biological features of eating disorders (Bulik et al., 2022). Current research is promising, but it's important to recognize that it is still in the early stages, and much additional work must be done before advances in neuroscience and genetics lead to direct clinical applications of research findings.

One advancement that appears especially promising is neuromodulation, or the use of procedures that in some way inhibit, stimulate, alter, or regulate nervous system functioning, to treat eating disorders. A specific type of neuromodulation called RTMS, or repetitive TMS, may be beneficial for reducing symptoms of eating disorders. Repetitive TMS uses an electromagnetic coil to stimulate specific brain regions. While it is primarily used in the treatment of depression, recent research using repetitive TMS to treat severe, enduring anorexia nervosa has revealed that it is effective for improving mood and quality of life, and it has small, albeit beneficial, effects on BMI and eating disorder symptoms. There is some evidence that repetitive TMS may reduce binge-eating and purging in bulimia nervosa, but there is a lack of research evaluating this intervention in binge-eating disorder. As neuroscience research expands, experts may discover which specific brain regions implicated in eating disorders should be the target of neuromodulation techniques (Gallop et al., 2022).

Digital and Technological Interventions

As technology advances, there has been growing interest in the use of digital and technological tools for the treatment of eating disorders. These interventions are often standalone treatments, and patients receive minimal to no therapist support while participating. They may be provided using SmartPhone apps or Internet websites, for example. A recent meta-analysis reviewed the results of research with digital interventions informed by behavioral change theory. These interventions help patients with eating disorders to change behaviors associated with disordered eating and replace them with new, healthier behaviors. According to the results of meta-analysis, interventions that allowed for self-monitoring of behavior were part of all effective interventions. Other techniques present in effective interventions included problem-solving, action planning, and learning about antecedents of behavior. This finding suggests that digital interventions based on behavioral theory can be effective for treating symptoms of eating disorders (Thomas et al., 2024).

Another meta-analysis of technological interventions evaluated the effects of a variety of different modalities, including those aimed at both prevention and treatment of eating disorders. These interventions were delivered via Internet, CD-ROM, or phone app. Many prevention-based interventions included in the meta-analysis involved components of mindfulness and cognitive-behavioral therapy. Some interventions involved text-based coaching. Treatment-focused interventions used CBT-based modalities. Results of the meta-analysis revealed that prevention-based interventions were effective for reducing dietary restriction, internalization of the thin ideal, and concerns related to weight and shape. Treatment-focused interventions were found to be effective for bulimia nervosa and binge-eating disorder. However, there is a lack of research related to digital treatments for anorexia nervosa, presumably because the severity of the disorder makes face-to-face treatment preferred (Linardon et al., 2020).

Self-help interventions such as apps and Internet programs are not the only eating disorder treatments delivered via technology, as some patients may participate in Internet-based therapy. The expansion of technology allows therapists to connect with patients via web camera, so patients can access treatment from remote locations. Research does suggest that therapy provided via web camera can increase treatment access and improve eating disorder symptoms. Therapists providing virtual services must be aware of laws in their jurisdictions, including regulations related to whether a patient must be physically located in the state where the therapist is licensed in order for the therapist to be permitted to provide services (Sproch & Anderson, 2019).

The evidence base surrounding virtual therapy is growing. One recent trial analyzing a virtual intervention for patients with anorexia nervosa, ranging in age from 6 to 24, found that enhanced family-based treatment resulted in weight gain, reductions in eating disorder symptoms, and improvement in caregiver self-efficacy. This trial confirmed that family-based eating disorder interventions can be delivered virtually (Steinberg et al., 2023). Finally, one recent study found that a partial hospitalization program (PHP) delivered virtually for 5 hours per day, 5 days a week, was feasible to implement and comparable in effectiveness to an in-person program. The PHP involved four hours of group therapy and two coached meals per session; one day per week, patients received a session of individual therapy, family therapy, and nutrition therapy instead of the group meeting (Penwell et al., 2024).

Emerging research suggests that digital interventions, including virtual therapy, can be successful for reducing symptoms in patients with eating disorders. These interventions can increase treatment access for those who live in rural areas or who face financial barriers to seeking treatment. They may also be appropriate for people negatively affected by stigma, as these groups can access digital treatment from the privacy and convenience of home. While current research findings with digital interventions are promising, additional studies are warranted, especially for evaluating the effectiveness of apps. It's also essential to consider that technological interventions may not be appropriate for those with moderate to severe eating disorders, and there is a lack of research evaluating the long-term effects of technological interventions (Linardon et al., 2020; Thomas et al., 2024).

CONCLUSION

The future of evidence-based eating disorder treatment depends upon several critical improvements. First, researchers must show a commitment to increasing the evidence base surrounding effective interventions for historically underrepresented groups. Similarly, clinicians must be prepared to deliver culturally sensitive interventions to these groups (Goel et al., 2022; Sonneville & Lipson, 2018). Furthermore, research must evaluate treatment options for severe and enduring anorexia nervosa and seek to determine which evidence-based interventions are more effective for promoting long-term recovery (Miskovic-Wheatley et al., 2023; Wonderlich et al., 2020). Finally, it is essential for clinicians to make a commitment to utilizing evidence-based treatments, which may require modifications to curriculum within university programs that educate future clinicians (Kazdin et al., 2017; Author, 2025). As researchers and clinicians seek to make the aforementioned improvements, emerging treatments, such as neuromodulation and digital interventions may play an increasingly essential role in the field of eating disorder treatment (Gallop et al., 2022; Thomas et al., 2024).

REFERENCES

Ben-Porath, D., Duthu, F., Luo, T., Gonidakis, F., Compte, E. J., & Wisniewski, L. (2020). Dialectical behavior therapy: An update and review of the existing treatment models adapted for adults with eating disorders. *Eating Disorders*, *28*(2), 101–121. DOI: 10.1080/10640266.2020.1723371 PMID: 32129724

Brockmeyer, T., Friederich, H. C., & Schmidt, U. (2018). Advances in the treatment of anorexia nervosa: A review of established and emerging interventions. *Psychological Medicine*, *48*(8), 1228–1256. DOI: 10.1017/S0033291717002604 PMID: 28889819

Gallop, L., Flynn, M., Campbell, I. C., & Schmidt, U. (2022). Neuromodulation and eating disorders. *Current Psychiatry Reports*, *24*(1), 61–69. DOI: 10.1007/s11920-022-01321-8 PMID: 35179712

Goel, N. J., Mathis, K. J., Egbert, A. H., Petterway, F., Breithaupt, L., Eddy, K. T., Franko, D. L., & Graham, A. K. (2022). Accountability in promoting representation of historically marginalized racial and ethnic populations in the eating disorders field: A call to action. *International Journal of Eating Disorders*, *55*(4), 463–469. DOI: 10.1002/eat.23682 PMID: 35092322

Kazdin, A. E., Fitzsimmons-Craft, E. E., & Wilfley, D. E. (2017). Addressing critical gaps in the treatment of eating disorders. *International Journal of Eating Disorders*, *50*(3), 170–189. DOI: 10.1002/eat.22670 PMID: 28102908

Linardon, J., Shatte, A., Messer, M., Firth, J., & Fuller-Tyszkiewicz, M. (2020). E-mental health interventions for the treatment and prevention of eating disorders: An updated systematic review and meta-analysis. *Journal of Consulting and Clinical Psychology*, *88*(11), 994–1007. DOI: 10.1037/ccp0000575 PMID: 32852971

MacCaughelty, C. R. (2023). Eating disorder mental health literacy: A national survey of clinical social workers in the United States. *Journal of Social Work : JSW*, *23*(2), 267–285. DOI: 10.1177/14680173221144217

Miskovic-Wheatley, J., Bryant, E., Ong, S. H., Vatter, S., Le, A., Aouad, P., Barakat, S., Boakes, R., Brennan, L., Bryant, E., Byrne, S., Caldwell, B., Calvert, S., Carroll, B., Castle, D., Caterson, I., Chelius, B., Chiem, L., Clarke, S., & Maguire, S.National Eating Disorder Research Consortium. (2023). Eating disorder outcomes: Findings from a rapid review of over a decade of research. *Journal of Eating Disorders*, *11*(85), 85. Advance online publication. DOI: 10.1186/s40337-023-00801-3 PMID: 37254202

Moreno, R., Buckelew, S. M., Accurso, E. C., & Raymond-Flesch, M. (2023). Disparities in access to eating disorders treatment for publicly-insured youth and youth of color: A retrospective cohort study. *Journal of Eating Disorders*, *11*(10), 10. Advance online publication. DOI: 10.1186/s40337-022-00730-7 PMID: 36694235

Nagata, J. M., Ganson, K. T., & Austin, S. B. (2020). Emerging trends in eating disorders among sexual and gender minorities. *Current Opinion in Psychiatry*, *33*(6), 562–567. DOI: 10.1097/YCO.0000000000000645 PMID: 32858597

Penwell, T. E., Bedard, S. P., Eyre, R., & Levinson, C. A. (2024). Eating disorder treatment access in the United States: Perceived inequities among treatment seekers. *Psychiatric Services (Washington, D.C.)*, *75*(10), 944–952. Advance online publication. DOI: 10.1176/appi.ps.20230193 PMID: 38716514

Penwell, T. E., Smith, M., Ortiz, S. N., Brooks, G., & Thompson-Brenner, H. (2024). Traditional versus virtual partial hospital programme for eating disorders: Feasibility and preliminary comparison of effects. *European Eating Disorders Review*, *32*(2), 163–178. DOI: 10.1002/erv.3031 PMID: 37677002

Rodgers, R. F., Berry, R., & Franko, D. L. (2018). Eating disorders in ethnic minorities: An update. *Current Psychiatry Reports*, *20*(90), 90. Advance online publication. DOI: 10.1007/s11920-018-0938-3 PMID: 30155577

Smith, J. (2023). A call to shift theoretical orientation for eating disorder treatment in social work: Inside-out and outside-in. *Health & Social Work*, *48*(4), 281–284. DOI: 10.1093/hsw/hlad019 PMID: 37608569

Sonneville, K. R., & Lipson, S. K. (2018). Disparities in eating disorder diagnosis and treatment according to weight status, race/ethnicity, socioeconomic background, and sex among college students. *International Journal of Eating Disorders, 51*(6), 518–526. DOI: 10.1002/eat.22846 PMID: 29500865

Sproch, L. E., & Anderson, K. P. (2019). Clinician-delivered teletherapy for eating disorders. *The Psychiatric Clinics of North America, 42*(2), 243–252. DOI: 10.1016/j.psc.2019.01.008 PMID: 31046926

Steinberg, D., Perry, T., Freestone, D., Bohon, C., Baker, J. H., & Parks, E. (2023). Effectiveness of delivering evidence-based eating disorder treatment via telemedicine for children, adolescents, and youth. *Eating Disorders, 31*(1), 85–101. DOI: 10.1080/10640266.2022.2076334 PMID: 35695470

Thomas, P. C., Curtis, K., Potts, H. W. W., Bark, P., Perowne, R., Rookes, T., & Rowe, S. (2024). Behavior change techniques within digital interventions for the treatment of eating disorders: Systematic review and meta-analysis. *JMIR Mental Health, 11*, e57577. DOI: 10.2196/57577 PMID: 39088817

White, M., Thomas, A., Aston, M., & Joy, P. (2024). "It's beautiful and it's messy and it's tragic": Exploring the role of compassion in the eating disorder recovery processes of 2S/LGBTQ+ Canadians. *Journal of Eating Disorders, 12*(23), 23. Advance online publication. DOI: 10.1186/s40337-024-00981-6 PMID: 38326869

Wonderlich, S. A., Bulik, C. M., Schmidt, U., Steiger, H., & Hoek, H. W. (2020). Achieving global impact: Increasing access to care and reducing the burden of eating disorders. *International Journal of Eating Disorders, 53*(8), 1303–1312. DOI: 10.1002/eat.23283 PMID: 32359125

KEY TERMS AND DEFINITIONS

JEDI: A model from the Eating Disorders Research Society that emphasizes justice, equity, diversity, and inclusion, to ensure that eating disorders research includes diverse participants from underrepresented groups

Neuromodulation: Treatment procedures that involve some sort of inhibiting, stimulation, alteration, or regulation of nervous system functioning

Repetitive TMS: A specific neuromodulation technique that uses an electromagnetic coil to stimulate certain regions of the brain

Research-Practice Gap: A phrase that refers to the fact that there is a gap between what is known about evidence-based treatment and the type of treatment eating disorder clinicians actually deliver

SE-AN: An acronym for severe and enduring anorexia nervosa, a presentation of the disorder in which a patient shows symptoms for over three years, and symptoms do not improve after participating in two evidence-based treatments

Chapter 15
Clinical Concepts Quick Guide

ABSTRACT

As the last chapter in this text, this chapter provides an overview of the key clinical concepts discussed throughout the text. This includes discussion of eating disorder assessment and diagnosis, risk factors for eating disorders, a brief review of evidence-based treatments, and description of specific therapeutic modalities used in eating disorder treatment. This chapter serves as a review of the most critical concepts addressed in the text, as well as a quick reference for someone seeking information.

INTRODUCTION

This text has covered a variety of topics related to evidence-based eating disorder assessment and intervention, beginning with an overview of eating disorder diagnosis and risk factors, before discussing the history of treatment and the current evidence base for eating disorder interventions. Next, the text discussed numerous evidence-based interventions, including individual, family, and group-based therapies. Final chapters in the textbook discussed levels of care, members of the eating disorder treatment team, cultural factors relevant to treatment, and the future of eating disorder treatment. This chapter concludes the text, providing a brief reference guide for clinical topics relevant to eating disorder treatment. It is useful for reviewing the core concepts presented in the textbook, or

DOI: 10.4018/979-8-3373-0664-3.ch015

for quickly finding information about a specific therapeutic modality or concept central to the treatment of eating disorders.

DIAGNOSTIC OVERVIEW AND ASSESSMENT STRATEGIES

Eating disorders are characterized by persistent disturbances in eating behaviors or related thoughts that result in health risks or functional impairment (APA, 2022). Core diagnoses include:

- **Anorexia Nervosa (AN):** Marked by restriction of energy intake, intense fear of gaining weight, and disturbance in self-perception of body weight or shape.
- **Bulimia Nervosa (BN):** Characterized by recurrent binge-eating episodes followed by compensatory behaviors such as vomiting or excessive exercise.
- **Binge-Eating Disorder (BED):** Involves recurrent episodes of binge eating without compensatory behaviors.
- **Avoidant/Restrictive Food Intake Disorder (ARFID):** Characterized by eating disturbances that result in nutritional deficiencies or dependence on supplements.
- **Pica:** An eating disorder in which a person repeatedly eats non-food substances that offer no nutritional value
- **Rumination Disorder:** Involves repeated regurgitation of food
- **Other Specified Feeding or Eating Disorder:** Diagnosed when a person does not meet criteria for another eating disorder and the clinician specifies why the criteria for another disorder are not met
- **Unspecified Feeding or Eating Disorder:** Diagnosed when a person does not meet criteria for another eating disorder and the clinician does not specific why the criteria for another disorder are not met

Assessment tools such as the **Eating Disorder Examination (EDE)** and **Eating Disorder Inventory (EDI)** help identify diagnostic features. Clinicians also use interviews, food diaries, BMI calculation, and medical assessments to determine illness severity and guide level of care decisions (APA, 2022).

The **SCOFF** (Morgan et al., 1999) is a simple, valid tool used in the identification of eating disorders (Kutz et al., 2020). This tool askes the following three questions:

1. Do you make yourself sick because you feel uncomfortably full?
2. Do you worry you have lost control over how much you eat?
3. Have you recently lost more than one stone in a 3-month period?
4. Would you say that food dominates your life?

RISK FACTORS FOR EATING DISORDERS

Risk factors for eating disorders are multifaceted and vary based on the type of eating disorder. Some of the main risk factors for the different eating disorders are highlighted below.

Risk Factors for Anorexia Nervosa

There are numerous factors that increase the risk of anorexia nervosa. The key risk factors for this disorder, based on the work of multiple authors, are listed below (Barakat et al., 2023; Batista et al., 2018; Dane & Bhatia, 2023; Del Casale et al., 2023; Haynos et al., 2016; Hilbert et al., 2014; Izydorczyk et al., 2020; Steinhausen et al., 2015; Stice et al., 2017; Van Dyne et al., 2023):

- Family-related risk factors, such as relational trauma, family history of psychiatric disorders, family expectations of perfectionism, family dysfunction and conflict, emotional issues in the family, low level of family involvement, demanding or problem parenting, parental substance use disorder, parenting (especially maternal) dieting, and poor family communication
- Genetics
- Low self-esteem
- Depressive symptoms

- Body dissatisfaction during childhood
- Perfectionist personality traits
- Psychological maladjustment
- Problems with emotion dysregulation
- Interpersonal problems
- Sociocultural pressures related to thinness
- Exposure to the thin ideal via social media
- Intergenerational trauma related to acculturation
- Dieting

Risk Factors for Bulimia Nervosa

Like anorexia nervosa, there are numerous risk factors for bulimia nervosa, based on the existing research (Barakat et al., 2023; Donato et al., 2022; Hilbert et al., 2014; Izydorczyk et al., 2020; Jakovina et al., 2018; Ruchkin et al., 2021; Van Dyne et al., 2023; Yamamiya & Stice, 2024; Zanella & Lee, 2022):

- Family-related factors, including low parental support, trauma, child maltreatment, family disruption, poor parenting skills, demanding parenting, family conflict, dieting and overeating within the family, family history of bulimia nervosa
- Genetics
- History of conduct problems
- History of childhood obesity
- Perfectionism
- Internalization of thin ideals and pressure to be thin
- Body dissatisfaction
- Co-occurring psychiatric disorders, including depression and anxiety
- Emotion regulation difficulties
- Attachment anxiety
- Acculturation and intergenerational trauma, especially in indigenous populations
- Being White compared to Black
- Using the media to obtain information about body standards

Risk Factors for Binge-Eating Disorder

The body of research has revealed the following risk factors associated with binge-eating disorder (Hilbert et al., 2014; Keski-Rahkonen, 2021; Rodgers et al., 2018; Steiger & Booij, 2020; Stice et al., 2017):

- Family-related risk factors, including separation from a parent, family history of bulimia nervosa, parental absence or death, family overeating, family trauma
- Genetics
- High anxiety
- Impulsive traits
- Body dissatisfaction
- Substance misuse
- Internalization of the thin ideal
- History of pregnancy
- Severe childhood obesity
- Conduct problems
- History of being bullied or teased
- Negative emotionality
- Having a mental health problem, including a mood disorder
- Being of Latino/a ethnicity

Risk Factors for Other Eating Disorders

There is less research available on risk factors for pica, ARFID, and rumination disorder, but the following factors may increase the risk for one of these diagnoses (Dinkler et al., 2023; Hartmann, 2015; Jansen et al., 2017; Kozak et al., 2023; Lucarelli et al., 2018; Sader et al., 2025; Zimmerman & Fisher, 2017):

- Parental pressure to eat (primarily in ARFID)
- Maternal mental illness
- Dysfunctional interactions between mother and child
- Having an intellectual disability or autism spectrum disorder
- History of trauma, neglect, or separation from parents

- Genetic factors
- Gastrointestinal problems, food allergies, sensory aversions to food, and history of choking or vomiting with food (primarily in ARFID)
- Iron deficiency anemia, pregnancy, or malnutrition (primarily in pica)

HIGHLIGHTS OF SYSTEMATIC REVIEW OF EVIDENCE-BASED EATING DISORDER INTERVENTIONS

A systematic review of evidence-based treatments for eating disorders was conducted for inclusion in this textbook. The following points summarize the key findings of this review:

- Family-based therapy is evidence-based for adolescents with anorexia nervosa, while enhanced cognitive behavioral therapy (CBT-E) is the treatment of choice for adults with this disorder (Brockmeyer et al., 2018; Marcolini et al., 2024; Zipfel et al., 2015).
- CBT is beneficial for adults with bulimia nervosa, and family-based treatment is likely beneficial for youth with bulimia nervosa, but additional research is warranted (Hagan & Walsh, 2021; Hail & Le Grange, 2018).
- CBT appears to be the treatment of choice for binge-eating disorder, though interpersonal psychotherapy, pharmacological options like lisdexamfetamine, and behavioral weight loss programs can also be effective (Grilo & Juarascio, 2023; Hilbert et al., 2019; Palavras et al., 2021).
- ARFID is best treated through a combination of dietary, psychological, and family-based strategies that first address nutritional deficits, but there is limited evidence related to effective treatments for this disorder (Archibald & Bryant-Waugh, 2023; Shimshoni et al., 2020; Willmott et al., 2024).
- Behavioral strategies are the treatment of choice for rumination disorder and pica, but for pica, pharmacological and nutritional interventions may supplement behavioral interventions, especially when

a patient has iron deficiency anemia (Ganesan & Vasauskas, 2023; Moline et al., 2021; Sasegbon et al., 2022; Williams et al., 2022).

SPECIFIC INTERVENTIONS USED IN EATING DISORDER TREATMENT

Numerous interventions are utilized in eating disorder treatment. While evidence does favor some interventions over others, as described above, treatment is not one-size-fits all. So, any of the interventions below may be utilized in eating disorder treatment, based upon a patient's specific needs:

- **Behavioral Approaches:** Modalities based on behaviorism, a theory that argues people learn behavior and therefore can learn new behaviors. Includes the following interventions:
    - **Acceptance and commitment therapy (ACT):** A third-wave cognitive behavioral therapy that emphasizes psychological flexibility and mindfulness practices to promote acceptance of uncomfortable emotions, while helping people choose new, values-aligned behaviors (Manlick et al., 2013)
    - **Behavioral Weight Loss:** An intervention for binge-eating disorder that helps patients implemented lifestyle changes that lead to structured eating patterns, increased physical activity, and moderate calorie reduction (Forman et al., 2023)
    - **Exposure and response prevention:** A specific type of exposure therapy that involves exposing a person to a a feared item, such as an "off limits" food and then preventing them from engaging in an anxiety-related response (Butler & Heimberg, 2020)
    - **Mindfulness-based interventions:** Interventions that emphasize present-moment awareness and attunement (Roos et al., 2021)
- **Dialectical Behavior Therapy (DBT):** DBT is a skills-based therapy adapted for EDs, particularly for individuals with binge/purge behaviors. It is grounded in the **biosocial theory**, which posits that emotion dysregulation results from the interaction of biological

sensitivity and invalidating environments (Linehan & Wilks, 2015). Key concepts include:

  - **Core modules:** Mindfulness, emotion regulation, distress tolerance, and interpersonal effectiveness.
  - **Target behaviors:** Impulsivity, binge eating, purging, and emotional avoidance.

- **Enhanced Cognitive-Behavioral Therapy (CBT-E):** A version of cognitive behavioral therapy (CBT) designed for treatment of eating disorders, that addresses factors like perfectionism, interpersonal conflict, low self-esteem, and problems with tolerating moods, which are common in individuals with eating disorders (Hagan & Walsh, 2021; Zipfel et al., 2015). Related concepts include:
  - **Cognitive behavioral therapy for BN (CBT-B):** A version of CBT developed specifically for bulimia nervosa; based on belief that people diet due to weight and shape concerns, which eventually results in a cycle of binge-eating and purging (Hagan & Walsh, 2021)
  - **Cognitive distortions:** Negative or biased ways of thinking that contribute to psychopathology, per the CBT model (Chand et al., 2023; Curtiss et al., 2021)
- **Family-Based Treatment (FBT):** empowers parents to take charge of refeeding and behavior normalization for youth with anorexia nervosa. Key terms include:
  - **Externalization of the illness:** Separating the eating disorder from the adolescent to avoid blame.
  - **Three-phase model:** Phase I emphasizes parental control of eating; Phase II transitions eating responsibility to the adolescent; Phase III addresses identity and relapse prevention (Loeb & Le Grange, 2009).
- **Group Therapy:** Treatment that is provided in group format and offers therapeutic benefits, such as cohesion and universality. Some specific group types include (Corey et al., 2018):
  - **Psychoeducation groups**: Group interventions that provide essential information

- **Psychotherapy groups:** Group interventions provided to people who have a mental health diagnosis that significantly interferes with functioning

- **Interpersonal Psychotherapy (IPT):** IPT is structured around improving **interpersonal functioning**, and is especially relevant when eating disorder symptoms are linked to grief, role transitions, interpersonal disputes, or skill deficits (Murphy et al., 2012). Key concepts include:
  - **Interpersonal inventory:** A mapping of the patient's relational history and functioning.
  - **Focus areas:** Grief, interpersonal disputes, role transitions, interpersonal deficits.
- **Other Family-Focused Treatments:** While family-based treatment (FBT) is the treatment of choice for adolescents, there are other family-focused models:
  - **Emotion-focused therapy:** A family therapy model that helps parents become emotion coaches for their children, so the child can regulate emotions without turning to disordered eating behaviors (Lafrance Robinson et al., 2015)
  - **Family systems therapy**: The approach based on the work of Dr. Murray Bowen that emphasizes helping family members to become differentiated (Brown & Errington, 2024)
  - **Strategic family therapy:** A family therapy model that seeks to interrupt repetitive patterns of interaction that maintain presenting problems through the use of purposeful interventions (Wetchler & Hecker, 2015)
  - **Structural family therapy:** Salvador Minuchin's family therapy model that focuses on reorganizing the family structure to solve problems (Wetchler & Hecker, 2015)
- **Person-Centered Therapy**: A modality that emphasizes helping people achieve growth through unconditional positive regard and therapeutic empathy (Sue et al., 2017)
- **Psychodynamic Therapy:** A therapeutic model based on the work of Sigmund Freud, the father of psychoanalytic theory. This model emphasizes the role that unconscious thoughts and unresolved

childhood conflicts play in psychopathology. Key terms from this model include (Sue et al., 2017; Zerbe, 2015):

- **Countertransference:** The emotional reactions of a therapist to a patient.
- **Defense mechanisms:** Unconscious methods patients use to keep painful information out of conscious awareness.
- **Free association:** The process of saying whatever comes to mind in order to help with identifying material in the subconscious.
- **Transference:** Instances in which the patient's behavior toward the therapist reflects experiences the patient has had in past relationships.

MULTIDISCIPLINARY TREATMENT AND LEVELS OF CARE

Eating disorder treatment is most effective with **interdisciplinary collaboration**. Roles include:

- **Therapists and social workers:** Deliver psychotherapy, facilitate care coordination.
- **Registered dietitians:** Guide nutritional rehabilitation and meal planning.
- **Physicians and nurses:** Monitor vitals, manage refeeding, and address medical complications.
- **Psychiatrists:** Evaluate and manage comorbid conditions and psychotropic medications.

Levels of care include:

- **Outpatient (OP):** Weekly sessions with therapist and dietitian.
- **Intensive Outpatient Program (IOP):** Approximately 9–12 hours/week of structured therapy and meal support.
- **Partial Hospitalization Program (PHP):** Full-day programming without overnight stay.

- **Residential and inpatient:** For clients requiring 24-hour supervision, typically due to medical or psychiatric instability (Lock & Le Grange, 2015).

CULTURAL COMPETENCE AND ADAPTATIONS

Effective ED treatment requires attention to **cultural identity**, **stigmatization**, and **disparities in access**. Examples from this textbook include:

- **Latina women:** Cultural values such as familism may influence engagement; inclusion of family members can improve retention and outcomes (Reyes-Rodriguez et al., 2014).
- **2S/LGBTQ+ clients:** Reports of being misunderstood or invalidated in traditional ED settings call for affirming, inclusive approaches (White et al., 2024).

Clinicians are encouraged to use the **Cultural Formulation Interview (CFI)** and remain aware of how systemic inequities and cultural norms impact symptom expression, diagnosis, and treatment adherence (APA, 2022).

REFERENCES

American Psychiatric Association. (2022). *Diagnostic and statistical manual of mental disorders* (5th ed., text rev.)., DOI: 10.1176/appi.books.9780890425787

Archibald, T., & Bryant-Waugh, R. (2023). Current evidence for avoidant restrictive food intake disorder: Implications for clinical practice and future directions. *JCPP Advances*, *3*(2), e12160. DOI: 10.1002/jcv2.12160 PMID: 37753149

Barakat, S., McLean, S. A., Bryant, E., Le, E., Marks, P., Touyz, S., & Maguire, S. (2023). Risk factors for eating disorders: Findings from a rapid review. *Journal of Eating Disorders*, *11*(8), 1–31. DOI: 10.1186/s40337-022-00717-4 PMID: 36650572

Batista, M., Žigić Antić, L., Žaja, O., Jakovina, T., & Begovac, I. (2018). Predictors of eating disorder risk in anorexia nervosa adolescents. *Acta Clinica Croatica*, *57*(3), 399–410. DOI: 10.20471/acc.2018.57.03.01 PMID: 31168171

Brockmeyer, T., Friederich, H. C., & Schmidt, U. (2018). Advances in the treatment of anorexia nervosa: A review of established and emerging interventions. *Psychological Medicine*, *48*(8), 1228–1256. DOI: 10.1017/S0033291717002604 PMID: 28889819

Brown, J., & Errington, L. (2024). Bowen family systems theory and practice: Illustration and critique revisited. *Australian and New Zealand Journal of Family Therapy*, *45*(2), 135–155. DOI: 10.1002/anzf.1589

Butler, R. M., & Heimberg, R. G. (2020). Exposure therapy for eating disorders: A systematic review. *Clinical Psychology Review*, *78*, 101851. DOI: 10.1016/j.cpr.2020.101851 PMID: 32224363

Chand, S. P., Kuckel, D. P., & Huecker, M. R. (2023). Cognitive behavior therapy. In *StatPearls*. StatPearls Publishing., https://www.ncbi.nlm.nih.gov/books/NBK470241/

Corey, M., Corey, G., & Corey, C. (2018). *Groups: Process and practice* (10th ed.). Cengage.

Curtiss, J. E., Levine, D. S., Ander, I., & Baker, A. W. (2021). Cognitive-behavioral treatments for anxiety and stress-related disorders. *Focus (San Francisco, Calif.), 19*(2), 142–149. DOI: 10.1176/appi.focus.20200045 PMID: 34690581

Dane, A., & Bhatia, K. (2023). The social media diet: A scoping review to investigate the association between social media, body image, and eating disorders amongst young people. *PLOS Global Public Health, 3*(3), e0001091. DOI: 10.1371/journal.pgph.0001091 PMID: 36962983

Del Casale, A., Adriani, B., Modesti, M. N., Virzi, S., Parmigiani, G., Vento, A. E., & Speranza, A. M. (2023). Anorexia nervosa and familial risk factors: A systematic review of the literature. *Current Psychology (New Brunswick, N.J.), 42*(29), 25476–25484. DOI: 10.1007/s12144-022-03563-4

Dinkler, L., Wronski, M.-L., Lichtenstein, P., Lundström, S., Larsson, H., Micali, N., Taylor, M. J., & Bulik, C. M. (2023). Etiology of the broad avoidant restrictive food intake disorder phenotype in Swedish twins aged 6 to 12 years. *JAMA Psychiatry, 80*(3), 260–269. DOI: 10.1001/jamapsychiatry.2022.4612 PMID: 36723946

Donato, K., Ceccarini, M. R., Dhuli, K., Bonetti, G., Medori, M. C., Marceddu, G., Precone, V., Xhufi, S., Bushati, M., Bozo, D., Beccari, T., & Bertelli, M. (2022). Gene variants in eating disorders: Focus on anorexia nervosa, bulimia nervosa, and binge-eating disorder. *Journal of Preventive Medicine and Hygiene, 63*(2, Suppl 3), E297–E305. DOI: 10.15167/2421-4248/jpmh2022.63.2S3.2772 PMID: 36479493

Forman, E. M., Evans, B. C., Berry, M. P., Lampe, E. W., Chwyl, C., & Zhang, F. (2023). Behavioral weight loss outcomes in individuals with binge-eating disorder: A meta-analysis. *Obesity (Silver Spring, Md.), 31*(8), 1981–1995. DOI: 10.1002/oby.23790 PMID: 37475687

Ganesan, P. R., & Vasauskas, A. A. (2023). The association between pica and iron-deficiency anemia: A scoping review. *Cureus, 15*(4), e37904. DOI: 10.7759/cureus.37904 PMID: 37220446

Grilo, C. M., & Juarascio, A. (2023). Binge-eating disorder interventions: Review, current status, and implications. *Current Obesity Reports*, *12*(3), 406–416. DOI: 10.1007/s13679-023-00517-0 PMID: 37439970

Hagan, K. E., & Walsh, B. T. (2021). State of the art: The therapeutic approaches to bulimia nervosa. *Clinical Therapeutics*, *43*(1), 40–49. DOI: 10.1016/j.clinthera.2020.10.012 PMID: 33358256

Hail, L., & Le Grange, D. (2018). Bulimia nervosa in adolescents: Prevalence and treatment challenges. *Adolescent Health, Medicine and Therapeutics*, *9*, 11–16. DOI: 10.2147/AHMT.S135326 PMID: 29379324

Hartmann, A. S. (2015). Pica and rumination disorder. In *Encyclopedia of Feeding and Eating Disorders* (pp. 1–5). Springer., DOI: 10.1007/978-981-287-087-2_40-1

Haynos, A. F., Watts, A. W., Loth, K. A., Pearson, C. M., & Neumark-Stzainer, D. (2016). Factors predicting an escalation of restrictive eating during adolescence. *The Journal of Adolescent Health*, *59*(4), 391–396. DOI: 10.1016/j.jadohealth.2016.03.011 PMID: 27161416

Hilbert, A., Petroff, D., Herpertz, S., Pietrowsky, R., Tuschen-Caffier, B., Vocks, S., & Schmidt, R. (2019). Meta-analysis of the efficacy of psychological and medical treatments for binge-eating disorder. *Journal of Consulting and Clinical Psychology*, *87*(1), 91–105. DOI: 10.1037/ccp0000358 PMID: 30570304

Hilbert, A., Pike, K. M., Goldschmidt, A. B., Wilfley, D. E., Fairburn, C. G., Dohm, F. A., Walsh, T., & Striegel Weissman, R. (2014). Risk factors across the eating disorders. *Psychiatry Research*, *220*(1-2), 500–506. DOI: 10.1016/j.psychres.2014.05.054 PMID: 25103674

Izydorczyk, B., Sitnik-Warchulska, K., Lizińczyk, S., & Lipowska, M. (2020). Socio-cultural standards promoted by the mass media as predictors of restrictive and bulimic behavior. *Frontiers in Psychiatry*, *11*, 506. DOI: 10.3389/fpsyt.2020.00506 PMID: 32581880

Jakovina, T., Crnković Batista, M., Ražić Pavičić, A., Žurić Jakovina, I., & Begovac, I. (2018). Emotional dysregulation and attachment dimensions in female patients with bulimia nervosa. *Psychiatria Danubina, 30*(1), 72–78. DOI: 10.24869/psyd.2018.72 PMID: 29546861

Jansen, P. W., de Barse, L. M., Jaddoe, V. W. V., Verhulst, F. C., Franco, O. H., & Tiemeier, H. (2017). Bi-directional associations between child fussy eating and parents' pressure to eat: Who influences whom? *Physiology & Behavior, 176*, 101–106. DOI: 10.1016/j.physbeh.2017.02.015 PMID: 28215424

Keski-Rahkonen, A. (2021). Epidemiology of binge eating disorder: Prevalence, course, comorbidity, and risk factors. *Current Opinion in Psychiatry, 34*(6), 525–531. DOI: 10.1097/YCO.0000000000000750 PMID: 34494972

Kozak, A., Czepczor-Bernat, K., Modrzejewska, J., Modrzejewska, A., Matusik, E., & Matusik, P. (2023). Avoidant/Restrictive Food Disorder (ARFID), food neophobia, other eating-related behaviours and feeding practices among children with autism spectrum disorder and in non-clinical sample: A preliminary study. *International Journal of Environmental Research and Public Health, 20*(10), 5822. DOI: 10.3390/ijerph20105822 PMID: 37239549

Kutz, A. M., Marsh, A. G., Gunderson, C. G., Maguen, S., & Masheb, R. M. (2020). Eating disorder screening: A systematic review and meta-analysis of diagnostic test characteristics of the SCOFF. *Journal of General Internal Medicine, 35*(3), 885–893. DOI: 10.1007/s11606-019-05478-6 PMID: 31705473

Lafrance Robinson, A., Dolhanty, J., & Greenberg, L. (2015). Emotion-focused family therapy for eating disorders in children and adolescents. *Clinical Psychology & Psychotherapy, 22*(1), 75–82. DOI: 10.1002/cpp.1861 PMID: 23913713

Linehan, M. M., & Wilks, C. R. (2015). The course and evolution of dialectical behavior therapy. *American Journal of Psychotherapy, 69*(2), 97–110. DOI: 10.1176/appi.psychotherapy.2015.69.2.97 PMID: 26160617

Loeb, K. L., & Le Grange, D. (2009). Family-based treatment for adolescent eating disorders: Current status, new applications and future directions. *International Journal of Child and Adolescent Health*, *2*(2), 243–254. DOI: 10.1080/10640266.2010.509688 PMID: 20191109

Lucarelli, L., Sechi, C., Cimino, S., & Chatoor, I. (2018). Avoidant/Restrictive Food Intake Disorder: A longitudinal study of malnutrition and psychopathological risk factors from 2to 11 years of age. *Frontiers in Psychology*, *9*, 1608. DOI: 10.3389/fpsyg.2018.01608 PMID: 30233458

Manlick, C. F., Cochran, S. V., & Koon, J. (2013). Acceptance and commitment therapy for eating disorders: Rationale and literature review. *Journal of Contemporary Psychotherapy*, *43*(2), 115–122. DOI: 10.1007/s10879-012-9223-7

Marcolini, F., Ravaglia, A., Tempia Valenta, S., Bosco, G., Marconi, G., De Ronchi, D., & Atti, A. R. (2024). Severe enduring anorexia nervosa (SE-AN) treatment options and their effectiveness: A review of literature. *Journal of Eating Disorders*, *12*(48), 48. Advance online publication. DOI: 10.1186/s40337-024-01006-y PMID: 38654374

Moline, R., Hou, S., Chevrier, J., & Thomassin, K. (2021). A systematic review of the effectiveness of behavioural treatments for pica in youths. *Clinical Psychology & Psychotherapy*, *28*(1), 39–55. DOI: 10.1002/cpp.2491 PMID: 32628326

Morgan, J. F., Reid, F., & Lacey, J. H. (1999). The SCOFF questionnaire: Assessment of a new screening tool for eating disorders. *BMJ (Clinical Research Ed.)*, *319*(7223), 1467–1468. DOI: 10.1136/bmj.319.7223.1467 PMID: 10582927

Murphy, R., Straebler, S., Basden, S., Cooper, Z., & Fairburn, C. G. (2012). Interpersonal psychotherapy for eating disorders. *Clinical Psychology & Psychotherapy*, *19*(2), 150–158. DOI: 10.1002/cpp.1780 PMID: 22362599

Palavras, M. A., Hay, P., Mannan, H., da Luz, F. Q., Sainsbury, A., Touyz, S., & Claudino, A. M. (2021). Integrated weight loss and cognitive behavioural therapy (CBT) for the treatment of recurrent binge eating and high body mass index: A randomized controlled trial. *Eating and Weight Disorders, 26*(1), 249–262. DOI: 10.1007/s40519-020-00846-2 PMID: 31983019

Rodgers, R. F., Berry, R., & Franko, D. L. (2018). Eating disorders in ethnic minorities: An update. *Current Psychiatry Reports, 20*(10), 90. DOI: 10.1007/s11920-018-0938-3 PMID: 30155577

Roos, C. R., Sala, M., Kober, H., Vanzhula, I. A., & Levinson, C. A. (2021). Mindfulness-based interventions for eating disorders: The potential to mobilize multiple associative-learning change mechanisms. *International Journal of Eating Disorders, 54*(9), 1601–1607. DOI: 10.1002/eat.23564 PMID: 34061387

Ruchkin, V., Isaksson, J., Schwab-Stone, M., & Stickley, A. (2021). Prevalence and early risk factors for bulimia nervosa symptoms in inner-city youth: Gender and ethnicity perspectives. *Journal of Eating Disorders, 9*(1), 136. DOI: 10.1186/s40337-021-00479-5 PMID: 34674763

Sader, M., Weston, A., Buchan, K., Kerr-Gaffney, J., Gillespie-Smith, K., Sharpe, H., & Duffy, F. (2025). The co-occurrence of autism and avoidant/restrictive food intake disorder (ARFID): A prevalence-based meta-analysis. *International Journal of Eating Disorders, 58*(3), 473–488. Advance online publication. DOI: 10.1002/eat.24369 PMID: 39760303

Sasegbon, A., Hasan, S. S., Disney, B. R., & Vasant, D. H. (2022). Rumination syndrome: Pathophysiology, diagnosis and practical management. *Frontline Gastroenterology, 13*(5), 402–409. DOI: 10.1136/flgastro-2021-101856 PMID: 36046491

Shimshoni, Y., Silverman, W. K., & Lebowitz, E. R. (2020, October). SPACE-ARFID : A pilot trial of a novel parent-based treatment for avoidant/restrictive food intake disorder. *International Journal of Eating Disorders, 53*(10), 1623–1635. DOI: 10.1002/eat.23341

Steiger, H., & Booij, L. (2020). Eating disorders, heredity and environmental activation: Getting epigenetic concepts into practice. *Journal of Clinical Medicine*, *9*(5), 1332. DOI: 10.3390/jcm9051332 PMID: 32375223

Steinhausen, H. C., Jakobsen, H., Helenius, D., Munk-Jørgensen, P., & Strober, M. (2015). A nation-wide study of the family aggregation and risk factors in anorexia nervosa over three generations. *International Journal of Eating Disorders*, *48*(1), 1–8. DOI: 10.1002/eat.22293 PMID: 24777686

Stice, E., Gau, J. M., Rohde, P., & Shaw, H. (2017). Risk factors that predict future onset of each *DSM–5* eating disorder: Predictive specificity in high-risk adolescent females. *Journal of Abnormal Psychology*, *126*(1), 38–51. DOI: 10.1037/abn0000219 PMID: 27709979

Sue, D., Sue, D. W., Sue, D., & Sue, S. (2017). *Essentials of understanding abnormal behavior* (3rd ed.). Cengage.

Van Dyne, A., Washington, N., Villodas, M., & Cronan, T. (2023). Racial/ethnic differences in anorexia and bulimia diagnoses among U.S. college students. *Eating Behaviors*, *50*, 101779. DOI: 10.1016/j.eatbeh.2023.101779 PMID: 37418803

Wetchler, J. L., & Hecker, L. L. (2015). *An introduction to marriage and family therapy* (2nd ed.). Routledge.

Williams, F., Gibbs, S., & Addo, A. S. (2022). The assessment and management of pica in people with intellectual disability. *BJPsych Advances*, *28*(6), 391–400. DOI: 10.1192/bja.2022.24

Willmott, E., Dickinson, R., Hall, C., Sadikovic, K., Wadhera, E., Micali, N., Trompeter, N., & Jewell, T. (2024). A scoping review of psychological interventions and outcomes for avoidant and restrictive food intake disorder (ARFID). *International Journal of Eating Disorders*, *57*(1), 27–61. DOI: 10.1002/eat.24073 PMID: 37876356

Yamamiya, Y., & Stice, E. (2024). Risk factors that predict future onset of anorexia nervosa, bulimia nervosa, binge eating disorder, and purging disorder in adolescent girls. *Behavior Therapy*, *55*(4), 712–723. DOI: 10.1016/j.beth.2023.10.002 PMID: 38937045

Zanella, E., & Lee, E. (2022). Integrative review on psychological and social risk and prevention factors of eating disorders including anorexia nervosa and bulimia nervosa: Seven major theories. *Heliyon*, *8*(11), e11422. DOI: 10.1016/j.heliyon.2022.e11422 PMID: 36406673

Zerbe, K. (2015). Psychodynamic theory of eating disorders. In Smolak, L., & Levine, M. P. (Eds.), *The Wiley handbook of eating disorders*. Wiley-Blackwell., DOI: 10.1002/9781118574089.ch20

Zimmerman, J., & Fisher, M. (2017). Avoidant/restrictive food intake disorder (ARFID). *Current Problems in Pediatric and Adolescent Health Care*, *47*(4), 95–103. DOI: 10.1016/j.cppeds.2017.02.005 PMID: 28532967

Zipfel, S., Giel, K. E., Bulik, C. M., Hay, P., & Schmidt, U. (2015). Anorexia nervosa: Aetiology, assessment, and treatment. *The Lancet. Psychiatry*, *2*(12), 1099–1111. https://www.thelancet.com/journals/lanpsy/article/PIIS2215-0366(15)00356-9/fulltext. DOI: 10.1016/S2215-0366(15)00356-9 PMID: 26514083

Conclusion

As we conclude this exploration of evidence-based treatments for eating disorders, it becomes clear that no single approach can meet the diverse needs of all individuals affected by these complex and multifaceted conditions. While some interventions may emerge as superior to others for certain populations, treatment does not use a one-size-fits all approach. For instance, family-based treatment may be the first line of intervention for adolescents with anorexia nervosa, but that doesn't suggest that no other treatments can be beneficial. Furthermore, some patients may require adaptations to evidence-based approaches to meet cultural their needs. So, it is essential for eating disorder professionals to have knowledge of a variety of treatment approaches, so they can use clinical expertise to select the best modality for a patient's unique needs. Beyond having knowledge of specific therapeutic modalities, eating disorder professionals must also demonstrate cultural humility and a commitment to interdisciplinary collaboration.

Throughout this text, we have examined the theoretical foundations and practical applications of leading treatment modalities—ranging from psychodynamic and cognitive-behavioral therapies to family-based and group approaches. This has involved exploring the evidence base underlying specific modalities. We have explored both longstanding models and more emerging strategies, and emphasized the importance of tailoring interventions to individual presentations, identities, and readiness for change. Yet, even as our understanding of eating disorders continues to expand, significant gaps remain in access to care, treatment equity, and long-term outcomes. Too many individuals still suffer in silence, facing stigma, misdiagnosis, or inadequate support. These challenges demand continued inquiry, advocacy, and transformation within the mental health and medical systems.

The call to action is clear: clinicians, educators, researchers, and policymakers must work together to advance early identification, culturally responsive treatment, and sustained recovery support. As readers and future leaders in this field, you are invited to bring curiosity, compassion, and courage to your work. Challenge assumptions. Center patients' lived experiences. Pursue innovation. And above all, remember that recovery is possible.

This text is not an endpoint, but a foundation. Let it propel you forward in your journey to support those affected by eating disorders—with knowledge, empathy, and an unwavering commitment to recovery for all, including populations historically underrepresented in eating disorder research.

Appendix

RECOMMENDED ASSIGNMENTS AND LEARNING ACTIVITIES

Students may choose to complete one or more of the following activities to supplement their learning, or the course instructor may choose to utilize these activities as course assignments to evaluate student mastery of course concepts. These assignments are appropriate for evaluating overall mastery of course concepts and are appropriate as final papers, final exams, or some other form of signature assignment.

1. Create a fictitious case of a patient showing symptoms of one of the eating disorders. Describe the case in detail, and formulate a diagnosis, based on criteria in the DSM-5-TR. Then, propose an evidence-based intervention for the patient, and support your chosen intervention with at least 3 scholarly sources.
2. Consider the following case:
    a. Tamaj is a 23-year-old woman who has come to treatment due to concerns with eating and weight. Tamaj reports that she binge-eats three times per week, and after binges, she feels anxious about gaining weight, so she rids herself of the calories by taking laxatives and running until she is satisfied she has burned off the calories consumed. Tamaj is experiencing extreme distress related to her symptoms. She has begun to withdraw from friends, because she is spending so much time fixating on her eating habits. Between binges, Tamaj attempts to restrain herself from overeating, but she eventually does succumb to another binge, which causes anxiety,

because Tamaj is dissatisfied with her body and feels she needs to lose weight.

b. Based on the case, give a diagnosis for Tamaj, based on criteria in the DSM-5-TR, and justify the diagnosis.
c. Recommend an evidence-based intervention for Tamaj, supporting your recommendation with at least three scholarly sources.

3. Propose a research study related to a topic in eating disorder assessment or treatment. First, conduct a literature review that includes at least 5 scholarly sources, published within the last 5 years. Based on the literature review, identify a gap in the research and propose a study that fills that gap. Describe what research question you'd like to explore, how you'll carry out your study, and what you'd hope to learn from the results.
4. Imagine you're a behavioral health professional, and you've been tasked with delivering an eating disorders prevention program to a local high school. Based on existing research, design a prevention program and prepare a paper that describes the program. Include a description of the theoretical orientation of the program, the content covered in the program, and the objectives of the program. Use at least 5 scholarly sources to support your writing.
5. Consider the following case:
    a. Emily is a 19-year-old college sophomore majoring in biology. She was referred to the university counseling center by her academic advisor due to concerns about weight loss, lack of energy, and frequent class absences. Emily lives in a dormitory, has a 3.9 GPA, and is described by professors and peers as highly intelligent but socially withdrawn and extremely perfectionistic. At the intake session, Emily appears visibly underweight. She reports having lost "around 20 pounds" over the past four months. Her BMI is currently 16.4 (height: 5'6"; weight: 102 lbs). She attributes her weight loss to "eating clean" and exercising, but admits that her food intake has become very restricted. She eats roughly 600–800 calories per day and engages in daily exercise (about 90–120 minutes of cardio). She says she sometimes skips meals to punish herself for "eating too much the day before."

Emily acknowledges being "terrified" of gaining weight and frequently checks her body in the mirror. She reports a persistent internal voice criticizing her appearance and efforts. She denies binge eating or purging but admits to feeling lightheaded when standing and frequently being cold. She has stopped menstruating for the past 5 months. Her vital signs taken by the campus health center show a resting heart rate of 48 bpm and low blood pressure. Emily shows high anxiety about food, particularly eating in public, and avoids social events that involve meals. She denies suicidal ideation but admits that she often feels hopeless and overwhelmed, especially when her routines are disrupted. Her family lives several states away and she says they are "worried but don't understand."

This is Emily's first time seeking treatment for mental health concerns. She expresses ambivalence about recovery, stating: "I know I probably can't keep going like this, but I don't want to gain weight. I feel in control for once." Based on this case presentation, make a diagnosis and recommend a treatment plan for Emily.

b. Based on Emily's presentation, determine which level of care you believe is most appropriate at this time: inpatient hospitalization, residential treatment, partial outpatient program (PHP), intensive outpatient program (IOP), or standard outpatient therapy.
c. Prepare a 2-3 page paper that recommends a level of care for Emily, supporting your recommendation with clinical reasoning. Consider the professional guidelines discussed in the textbook. In addition to the textbook, cite 3 additional outside sources to support your decision. Consider factors such as medical stability, daily functioning, level of support in the environment, psychological symptoms, and nutritional status when making your placement decision.

MASTERY QUESTIONS

The questions below can be used for studying purposes to review for a course exam. Alternatively, a course instructor may choose to utilize some or all of these questions for exams or quizzes.

1. Which of the following is a key diagnostic criterion for anorexia nervosa in the DSM-5-TR?
   A. Episodes of purging after meals
   B. Marked restriction of energy intake leading to significantly low body weight
   C. Weight gain despite excessive exercise
   D. Eating large amounts of food in short periods
2. ARFID is distinct from other eating disorders because:
   A. It involves distorted body image.
   B. It leads to obesity.
   C. It is not motivated by body image concerns.
   D. It always results in purging behaviors.
3. Which of the following populations is disproportionately underdiagnosed for eating disorders?
   A. White adolescent girls
   B. People of color
   C. Children under five
   D. Elderly adults
4. Early psychoanalytic approaches to eating disorders viewed symptoms as:
   A. Biological disturbances
   B. Culturally constructed patterns
   C. Manifestations of unconscious conflict
   D. Reactions to viral infections
5. What is considered the gold standard treatment for bulimia nervosa?
   A. ACT
   B. CBT-E
   C. FBT
   D. Nutritional counseling

6. Which assessment tool would most likely be used to evaluate eating disorder symptoms?
   A. Beck Depression Inventory
   B. The SCOFF
   C. Child Behavior Checklist
   D. Mood Disorder Questionnaire
7. Which diagnosis below would be most likely for a person who bases self-worth on weight and body shape and engages in binge-eating episodes, followed by purging, at least 3 times per week?
   A. Bulimia Nervosa
   B. Anorexia Nervosa
   C. Binge-Eating Disorder
   D. Other Specified Feeding or Eating Disorder
8. Which of the following would be the most appropriate placement for a patient who is medically stable but demonstrates severe symptoms of anorexia nervosa that are difficult for the patient to control without around-the-clock monitoring and structure?
   A. Inpatient Hospitalization
   B. Residential Treatment
   C. Intensive Outpatient Treatment (IOP)
   D. Standard Outpatient Treatment
9. What is the primary difference between bulimia nervosa and binge-eating disorder?
   A. Binge-eating disorder is the current name for what used to be binge-eating disorder.
   B. Bulimia nervosa is only diagnosed in adults, whereas binge-eating disorder can be diagnosed in children.
   C. Individuals with binge-eating disorder do not purge after binge-eating episodes; whereas individuals with bulimia nervosa engage in inappropriate purging after binge episodes.
   D. Individuals with bulimia nervosa must be underweight to be diagnosed, but there is no specification related to weight in diagnostic criteria for binge-eating disorder.
10. Which of the following best represents the psychodynamic view toward eating disorders?
   A. It views them as being linked to distorted thinking patterns.

B. It views them as arising from interpersonal deficits, such as grief, conflict, or inadequate social skills.
C. It argues they can be treated by teaching distress tolerance skills, mindfulness, emotion regulation, and interpersonal effectiveness.
D. It conceptualizes eating disorders as caused by disruptions in early attachment experiences and subconscious inner conflicts.

11. Which of the following eating disorder diagnoses would you most expect in a child who has iron deficiency anemia?
    A. Bulimia nervosa
    B. Binge-eating disorder
    C. Other specified feeding or eating disorder
    D. Pica
12. Which personality trait would you most expect in someone diagnosed with anorexia nervosa?
    A. Perfectionism
    B. Impulsivity
    C. Extreme extroversion
    D. Low conscientiousness
13. Which of the following treatments for adolescents with anorexia nervosa has the strongest evidence base?
    A. Family-based therapy
    B. Psychodynamic therapy
    C. Social skills training
    D. DBT skills groups
14. Which therapeutic modality is likely to explore social problems, like grief and relationship conflict?
    A. Cognitive Behavioral Therapy
    B. Interpersonal Psychotherapy
    C. Acceptance and Commitment Therapy
    D. Mindfulness-Based Interventions
15. Which of the following is not a core component of dialectical behavior therapy (DBT?)
    A. Skills groups
    B. Individual therapy
    C. Therapist group consultations
    D. Free association

16. Which of the following therapeutic modalities involves helping people to tolerate uncomfortable emotions while choosing new behaviors that align with their values?
    A. Interpersonal Psychotherapy
    B. Cognitive Behavioral Therapy
    C. Acceptance and Commitment Therapy
    D. Behavioral Weight Loss
17. Which of the following is a core component of cognitive behavioral therapy (CBT) as applied to eating disorders?
    A. Free association to explore unconscious material
    B. Cognitive restructuring to challenge distorted beliefs
    C. Externalization of the illness through parent-led refeeding
    D. Use of antipsychotic medication to reduce obsessive thoughts
18. Which group has historically been underrepresented in eating disorder research, contributing to disparities in treatment access and effectiveness?
    A. College-educated women
    B. Privately insured White adolescents
    C. LGBTQ+ individuals and racial/ethnic minorities
    D. Middle-aged male athletes
19. Which of the following is most accurate about long-term remission in anorexia nervosa?
    A. Most patients achieve full recovery within one year.
    B. Long-term remission rates are low.
    C. Relapse is rare in those who complete inpatient treatment.
    D. Most relapse occurs within the first month post-discharge.
20. According to recent research, which component is present in all effective digital interventions for eating disorders?
    A. Therapist-led daily video sessions
    B. Peer support forums
    C. Self-monitoring of eating behavior
    D. Calorie restriction protocols

COMPLETE ANSWER KEY

1. B
2. C
3. B
4. C
5. B
6. B
7. A
8. B
9. C
10. D
11. D
12. A
13. A
14. B
15. D
16. C
17. B
18. C
19. B
20. C

Compilation of References

Abbate-Daga, G., Marzola, E., Amianto, F., & Fassino, S. (2016). A comprehensive review of psychodynamic treatments for eating disorders. *Eating and Weight Disorders*, *21*(4), 553–580. DOI: 10.1007/s40519-016-0265-9 PMID: 26980319

Abdoli, M., Rosato, M. S., Desousa, A., & Cotrufo, P. (2024). Cultural differences in body image: A systematic review. *Social Sciences (Basel, Switzerland)*, *13*(6), 305. DOI: 10.3390/socsci13060305

Acle, A., Cook, B. J., & Beasley, T. (2021). Cultural considerations in the treatment of eating disorders among racial/ethnic minorities: A systematic review. *Journal of Cross-Cultural Psychology*, *52*(5), 379–399. DOI: 10.1177/00220221211017664

Agras, W. S., & Bohon, C. (2021). Cognitive behavioral therapy for the eating disorders. *Annual Review of Clinical Psychology*, *17*(1), 417–438. DOI: 10.1146/annurev-clinpsy-081219-110907 PMID: 33962536

Agras, W. S., Lock, J., Brandt, H., Bryson, S. W., Dodge, E., Halmi, K. A., Jo, B., Johnson, C., Kaye, W., Wilfley, D., & Woodside, B. (2014). Comparison of 2 family therapies for adolescent anorexia nervosa: A randomized parallel trial. *JAMA Psychiatry*, *71*(11), 1279–1286. DOI: 10.1001/jamapsychiatry.2014.1025 PMID: 25250660

American Nurses Association. (2015). *Code of ethics for nurses with interpretive statements* (2nd ed.). American Nurses Publishing.

American Psychiatric Association. (2016). *Feeding and eating disorders: DSM-5 selections*. American Psychiatric Association.

American Psychiatric Association. (2022). *Diagnostic and statistical manual of mental disorders* (5th ed., text rev.)., DOI: 10.1176/appi.books.9780890425787

American Psychiatric Association. (2023). *Practice guideline for the treatment of patients with eating disorders* (4th ed.)., DOI: 10.1176/appi.books.9780890425862

American Psychological Association. (2017). *Ethical principles of psychologists and code of conduct* (2002, Amended June 1, 2010, and January 1, 2017). https://www.apa.org/ethics/code

American Psychological Association. (2020, February 25). *Eating disorders: How psychotherapy can help people recover*. https://www.apa.org/topics/eating-disorders/psychotherapy

Amianto, F., Northoff, G., Abbate Daga, G., Fassino, S., & Tasca, G. A. (2016). Is anorexia nervosa a disorder of the self? A psychological approach. *Frontiers in Psychology*, *7*(849). Advance online publication. DOI: 10.3389/fpsyg.2016.00849 PMID: 27378967

Anderson, L. K., Reilly, E. E., Berner, L., Wierenga, C. E., Jones, M. D., Brown, T. A., Kaye, W. H., & Cusack, A. (2017). Treating eating disorders at higher levels of care: Overview and challenges. *Current Psychiatry Reports*, *19*(48), 48. Advance online publication. DOI: 10.1007/s11920-017-0796-4 PMID: 28653117

Archibald, T., & Bryant-Waugh, R. (2023). Current evidence for avoidant restrictive food intake disorder: Implications for clinical practice and future directions. *JCPP Advances*, *3*(2), e12160. DOI: 10.1002/jcv2.12160 PMID: 37753149

Assaz, D. A., Roche, B., Kanter, J. W., & Oshiro, C. K. B. (2018). Cognitive defusion in Acceptance and Commitment Therapy: What are the basic processes of change? *The Psychological Record*, *68*, 405–418. https://doi.org/10.1007/s40732-017-0254-z

Astrachan-Fletcher, E., Accurso, E. C., Rossman, S., McClanahan, S. F., Dimitropoulos, G., & Le Grange, D. (2018). An exploratory study of challenges and successes in implementing adapted family-based treatment in a community setting. *Journal of Eating Disorders*, *6*(44), 44. Advance online publication. DOI: 10.1186/s40337-018-0228-9 PMID: 30603086

Bankoff, S. M., Karpel, M. G., Forbes, H. E., & Pantalone, D. W. (2012). A systematic review of dialectical behavior therapy for the treatment of eating disorders. *Eating Disorders*, *20*(3), 196–215. DOI: 10.1080/10640266.2012.668478 PMID: 22519897

Barakat, S., McLean, S. A., Bryant, E., Le, E., Marks, P., Touyz, S., & Maguire, S. (2023). Risk factors for eating disorders: Findings from a rapid review. *Journal of Eating Disorders*, *11*(8), 1–31. DOI: 10.1186/s40337-022-00717-4 PMID: 36650572

Batista, M., Žigić Antić, L., Žaja, O., Jakovina, T., & Begovac, I. (2018). Predictors of eating disorder risk in anorexia nervosa adolescents. *Acta Clinica Croatica*, *57*(3), 399–410. DOI: 10.20471/acc.2018.57.03.01 PMID: 31168171

Bendall, C., & Taylor, N. F. (2023). The effect of oral refeeding compared with nasogastric refeeding on the quality of care for patients hospitalised with an eating disorder: A systematic review. *Nutrition & Dietetics: the Journal of the Dietitians Association of Australia*, *80*(1), 44–54. DOI: 10.1111/1747-0080.12770 PMID: 36254572

Ben-Porath, D., Duthu, F., Luo, T., Gonidakis, F., Compte, E. J., & Wisniewski, L. (2020). Dialectical behavior therapy: An update and review of the existing treatment models adapted for adults with eating disorders. *Eating Disorders*, *28*(2), 101–121. DOI: 10.1080/10640266.2020.1723371 PMID: 32129724

Bernecker, S. L., Coyne, A. E., Constantino, M. J., & Ravitz, P. (2017). For whom does interpersonal psychotherapy work? A systematic review. *Clinical Psychology Review*, *56*, 82–93. DOI: 10.1016/j.cpr.2017.07.001 PMID: 28710917

Berner, L. A., Winter, S. R., Ayaz, H., Shewokis, P. A., Izzetoglu, M., Marsh, R., Nasser, J. A., Matteucci, A. J., & Lowe, M. R. (2023). Altered prefrontal activation during the inhibition of eating responses in women with bulimia nervosa. *Psychological Medicine*, *53*(8), 3513–3523. DOI: 10.1017/S0033291722000198 PMID: 35209961

Binh, T. T. N., & Huong, X. V. (2024). Eating disorders: A historical perspective and analysis of current treatment approaches. *International Journal of Innovative Research in Multidisciplinary Education*, *3*(4), 513–519. DOI: 10.58806/ijirme.2024.v3i4n07

Bray, M., Heruc, G., Evans, L., & Wright, O. R. L. (2024). The imperative of collaboration: Lived experience perspectives on team approaches in outpatient eating disorder treatment. *International Journal of Eating Disorders*, *57*(1), 116–123. DOI: 10.1002/eat.24084 PMID: 37902406

Brockmeyer, T., Friederich, H. C., & Schmidt, U. (2018). Advances in the treatment of anorexia nervosa: A review of established and emerging interventions. *Psychological Medicine*, *48*(8), 1228–1256. DOI: 10.1017/S0033291717002604 PMID: 28889819

Brown, J., & Errington, L. (2024). Bowen family systems theory and practice: Illustration and critique revisited. *Australian and New Zealand Journal of Family Therapy*, *45*(2), 135–155. DOI: 10.1002/anzf.1589

Brown, T. A., Wisniewski, L., & Anderson, L. K. (2020). Dialectical behavior therapy for eating disorders: State of the research and new directions. *Eating Disorders*, *28*(2), 97–100. DOI: 10.1080/10640266.2020.1728204 PMID: 32301685

Butler, R. M., & Heimberg, R. G. (2020). Exposure therapy for eating disorders: A systematic review. *Clinical Psychology Review*, *78*, 101851. https://doi.org/10.1016/j.cpr.2020.101851

Calatrava, M., Martins, M. V., Schweer-Collins, M., Duch-Ceballos, C., & Rodríguez-González, M. (2022). Differentiation of self: A scoping review of Bowen Family Systems Theory's core construct. *Clinical Psychology Review*, *91*, 102101. Advance online publication. DOI: 10.1016/j.cpr.2021.102101 PMID: 34823190

Carmel, A., Rose, M., & Fruzzetti, A. E. (2014). Barriers and solutions to implementing dialectical behavior therapy in a public behavioral health system. *Administration and Policy in Mental Health*, *41*(5), 608–614. DOI: 10.1007/s10488-013-0504-6 PMID: 23754686

Chand, S. P., Kuckel, D. P., & Huecker, M. R. (2023). Cognitive behavior therapy. In *StatPearls*. StatPearls Publishing., https://www.ncbi.nlm.nih.gov/books/NBK470241/

Cheng, Z. H., Perko, V. L., Fuller-Marashi, L., Gau, J. M., & Stice, E. (2019). Ethnic differences in eating disorder prevalence, risk factors, and predictive effects of risk factors among young women. *Eating Behaviors*, *32*, 23–30. DOI: 10.1016/j.eatbeh.2018.11.004 PMID: 30529736

Chmiel, J., Gladka, A., & Leszek, J. (2023). The effect of transcranial direct current stimulation (tDCS) on anorexia nervosa: A narrative review. *Nutrients*, *15*(20), 4455. DOI: 10.3390/nu15204455 PMID: 37892530

Corey, M., Corey, G., & Corey, C. (2018). *Groups: Process and practice* (10th ed.). Cengage.

Crane, R. S., Brewer, J., Feldman, C., Kabat-Zinn, J., Santorelli, S., Williams, J. M. G., & Kuyken, W. (2017). What defines mindfulness-based programs? The warp and the weft. *Psychological Medicine*, *47*(6), 990–999. DOI: 10.1017/S0033291716003317

Cryan, J. F., & Dinan, T. G. (2012). Mind-altering microorganisms: The impact of the gut microbiota on brain and behaviour. *Nature Reviews. Neuroscience*, *13*(10), 701–712. DOI: 10.1038/nrn3346 PMID: 22968153

Cuerda, C., Vasiloglou, M. F., & Arhip, L. (2019). Nutritional management and outcomes in malnourished medical inpatients: Anorexia nervosa. *Journal of Clinical Medicine*, *8*(7), 1042. DOI: 10.3390/jcm8071042 PMID: 31319585

Curtiss, J. E., Levine, D. S., Ander, I., & Baker, A. W. (2021). Cognitive-behavioral treatments for anxiety and stress-related disorders. *Focus (San Francisco, Calif.)*, *19*(2), 142–149. DOI: 10.1176/appi.focus.20200045 PMID: 34690581 da Luz, F. Q., Hay, P., Wisniewski, L., Cordás, T., & Sainsbury, A. (2020). The treatment of binge eating disorder with cognitive behavior therapy and other therapies: An overview and clinical considerations. *Obesity Reviews*, *22*(5, S1), e13180. DOI: 10.1111/obr.13180 PMID: 33350574

Dane, A., & Bhatia, K. (2023). The social media diet: A scoping review to investigate the association between social media, body image, and eating disorders amongst young people. *PLOS Global Public Health*, *3*(3), e0001091. DOI: 10.1371/journal.pgph.0001091 PMID: 36962983

Davis, C. (2015). The epidemiology and genetics of binge eating disorder (BED). *CNS Spectrums*, *20*(6), 522–529. DOI: 10.1017/S1092852915000462 PMID: 26258270

Del Casale, A., Adriani, B., Modesti, M. N., Virzi, S., Parmigiani, G., Vento, A. E., & Speranza, A. M. (2023). Anorexia nervosa and familial risk factors: A systematic review of the literature. *Current Psychology (New Brunswick, N.J.)*, *42*(29), 25476–25484. DOI: 10.1007/s12144-022-03563-4

Delgado, S. V., Strawn, J. R., & Pedapati, E. (2015). *Contemporary psychodynamic psychotherapy for children and adolescents: Integrating intersubjectivity and neuroscience*. Springer. DOI: 10.1007/978-3-642-40520-4

Dell'Osso, L., Abelli, M., Carpita, B., Pini, S., Castellini, G., Carmassi, C., & Ricca, V. (2016).

Dinkler, L., Wronski, M.-L., Lichtenstein, P., Lundström, S., Larsson, H., Micali, N., Taylor, M. J., & Bulik, C. M. (2023). Etiology of the broad avoidant restrictive food intake disorder phenotype in Swedish twins aged 6 to 12 years. *JAMA Psychiatry*, *80*(3), 260–269. DOI: 10.1001/jamapsychiatry.2022.4612 PMID: 36723946

Donato, K., Ceccarini, M. R., Dhuli, K., Bonetti, G., Medori, M. C., Marceddu, G., Precone, V., Xhufi, S., Bushati, M., Bozo, D., Beccari, T., & Bertelli, M. (2022). Gene variants in eating disorders: Focus on anorexia nervosa, bulimia nervosa, and binge-eating disorder. *Journal of Preventive Medicine and Hygiene*, *63*(2, Suppl 3), E297–E305. DOI: 10.15167/2421-4248/jpmh2022.63.2S3.2772 PMID: 36479493

Dowd, E. T. (2004). Cognition and the cognitive revolution in psychotherapy: Promises and advances. *Journal of Clinical Psychology*, *60*(4), 415–428. DOI: 10.1002/jclp.10253 PMID: 15022271

Egbert, A. H., Hunt, R. A., Williams, K. L., Burke, N. L., & Mathis, K. J. (2022). Reporting racial and ethnic diversity in eating disorder research over the past 20 years. *International Journal of Eating Disorders*, *55*(4), 455–462. DOI: 10.1002/eat.23666 PMID: 34997609

Emelianchik-Key, K., Labarta, A., & Gill, C. S. (2023). The mediating role of transdiagnostic factors in a clinical sample of Black, Indigenous, and People of Color with eating disorders. *Journal of Mental Health Counseling*, *45*(4), 340–356. DOI: 10.17744/mehc.45.4.04

Farrell, E. (1995). Psychoanalytic understanding. In Young, R. M. (Ed.), *Lost for words: The psychoanalysis of anorexia and bulimia*. Psychoanalysis and Psychotherapy., Retrieved from https://www.psychoanalysis-and-therapy.com/human_nature/farrell/chap2.html

Fawcett, E. J., Fawcett, J. M., & Mazmanian, D. (2016). A meta-analysis of the worldwide prevalence of pica during pregnancy and the postpartum period. *International Journal of Gynaecology and Obstetrics: the Official Organ of the International Federation of Gynaecology and Obstetrics*, *133*(3), 277–283. DOI: 10.1016/j.ijgo.2015.10.012 PMID: 26892693

Fields, V. L., Soke, G. N., Reynolds, A., Tian, L. H., Wiggins, L., Maenner, M., DiGuiseppi, C., Kral, T. V. E., Hightshoe, K., & Schieve, L. A. (2021). Pica, autism, and other disabilities. *Pediatrics*, *147*(2), e20200462. DOI: 10.1542/peds.2020-0462 PMID: 33408069

Flanagan, L. M. (2021). The theory of self psychology. In Berzoff, J., Flanagan, L. M., & Hertz, P. (Eds.), *Inside out and outside in: Psychodynamic clinical theory and psychopathology in contemporary multicultural contexts* (5th ed., pp. 125–151). Rowman & Littlefield.

Fogelkvist, M., Gustafsson, S. A., Kjellin, L., & Parling, T. (2020). Acceptance and Commitment Therapy to reduce eating disorder symptoms and body image problems in patients with residual eating disorder symptoms: A randomized controlled trial. *Body Image*, *32*, 155–166. DOI: 10.1016/j.bodyim.2020.01.002

Forman, E. M., Evans, B. C., Berry, M. P., Lampe, E. W., Chwyl, C., & Zhang, F. (2023). Behavioral weight loss outcomes in individuals with binge-eating disorder: A meta-analysis. *Obesity (Silver Spring, Md.)*, *31*(8), 1981–1995. DOI: 10.1002/oby.23790

Friederich, H.-C., Zipfel, S., & Wild, B. (2023). Psychodynamic Therapies and Eating Disorders. In *Eating Disorders* (pp. 1–20). Springer., DOI: 10.1007/978-3-030-97416-9_66-1

Frostad, S., & Bentz, M. (2022). Anorexia nervosa: Outpatient treatment and medical management. *World Journal of Psychiatry*, *12*(4), 558–579. DOI: 10.5498/wjp.v12.i4.558 PMID: 35582333

Gabbard, G. O. (2004). *Long-term psychodynamic psychotherapy: A basic text*. American Psychiatric Publishing.

Gallop, L., Flynn, M., Campbell, I. C., & Schmidt, U. (2022). Neuromodulation and eating disorders. *Current Psychiatry Reports*, *24*(1), 61–69. DOI: 10.1007/s11920-022-01321-8 PMID: 35179712

Ganesan, P. R., & Vasauskas, A. A. (2023). The association between pica and iron-deficiency anemia: A scoping review. *Cureus*, *15*(4), e37904. DOI: 10.7759/cureus.37904 PMID: 37220446

Gioia, A. N., Morales, C., Laboe, A. A., Dolan, S. C., & Reilly, E. E. (2025). Clinical experiences using family based treatment for eating disorders. *International Journal of Eating Disorders*, *58*(4), 735–747. DOI: 10.1002/eat.24373 PMID: 39834197

Glasofer, D. R., Sysko, R., & Walsh, B. T. (2016). The use of the Eating Disorder Assessment for DSM-5 (EDA-5). In Sysko, R., Glasofer, D. R., Attia, E., & Walsh, B. T. (Eds.), *Handbook of Assessment and Treatment of Eating Disorders* (pp. 175–206). American Psychiatric Association.

Godfrey, K. M., Gallo, L. C., & Afari, N. (2015). Mindfulness-based interventions for binge eating: A systematic review and meta-analysis. *Journal of Behavioral Medicine*, *38*(2), 348–362. https://doi.org/10.1007/s10865-014-9610-5

Goel, N. J., Mathis, K. J., Egbert, A. H., Petterway, F., Breithaupt, L., Eddy, K. T., Franko, D. L., & Graham, A. K. (2022). Accountability in promoting representation of historically marginalized racial and ethnic populations in the eating disorders field: A call to action. *International Journal of Eating Disorders*, *55*(4), 463–469. DOI: 10.1002/eat.23682 PMID: 35092322

Goel, N. J., Thomas, B., Boutté, R. L., Kaur, B., & Mazzeo, S. E. (2023). "What will people say?": Mental health stigmatization as a barrier to eating disorder treatment-seeking for South Asian American women. *Asian American Journal of Psychology*, *14*(1), 96–113. DOI: 10.1037/aap0000271 PMID: 37283957

Goldman, R. N. (2019). History and overview of emotion-focused therapy. In L. S. DOI: 10.1037/0000112-001

Goodier, G. H. G., McCormack, J., Egan, S. J., Watson, H. J., Hoiles, K. J., & Byrne, S. M. (2014). Parent skills training treatment for parents of children and adolescents with eating disorders: A qualitative study. *International Journal of Eating Disorders*, *47*(4), 368–375. DOI: 10.1002/eat.22224 PMID: 24843891

Gordon, K. H., Brattole, M. M., Wingate, L. R., & Joiner, T. E.Jr. (2006). The impact of client race on clinician detection of eating disorders. *Behavior Therapy*, *37*(4), 319–325. DOI: 10.1016/j.beth.2005.12.002 PMID: 17071210

Gordon, K. H., Perez, M., & Joiner, T. E.Jr. (2002). The impact of racial stereotypes on eating disorder recognition. *International Journal of Eating Disorders, 32*(2), 219–224. DOI: 10.1002/eat.10070 PMID: 12210665

Gorrell, S., Reilly, E. E., Brosof, L., & Le Grange, D. (2022). Use of telehealth in the management of adolescent eating disorders: Patient perspectives and future directions suggested from the COVID-19 pandemic. *Adolescent Health, Medicine and Therapeutics, 13*, 45–53. DOI: 10.2147/AHMT.S334977 PMID: 35401019

Graves, L. (n.d). *Levels of care.* National Eating Disorders Association. Retrieved June 13, 2025, from https://www.nationaleatingdisorders.org/levels-of-care/

Grennan, L., Nicula, M., Pellegrini, D., Giuliani, K., Crews, E., Webb, C., Gouveia, M.-R., Loewen, T., & Couturier, J. (2022). "I'm not alone": A qualitative report of experiences among parents of children with eating disorders attending virtual parent-led peer support groups. *Journal of Eating Disorders, 10*(195), 195. Advance online publication. DOI: 10.1186/s40337-022-00719-2 PMID: 36522772

Grenon, R., Schwartze, D., Hammond, N., Ivanova, I., Mcquaid, N., Proulx, G., & Tasca, G. A. (2017). Group psychotherapy for eating disorders: A meta-analysis. *International Journal of Eating Disorders, 50*(9), 997–1013. DOI: 10.1002/eat.22744 PMID: 28771758

Grilo, C. M. (2017). Psychological and behavioral treatments for binge-eating disorder. *The Journal of Clinical Psychiatry, 78*(Suppl 1), 20–24. DOI: 10.4088/JCP.sh16003su1c.04 PMID: 28125175

Grilo, C. M., & Juarascio, A. (2023). Binge-eating disorder interventions: Review, current status, and implications. *Current Obesity Reports, 12*(3), 406–416. DOI: 10.1007/s13679-023-00517-0 PMID: 37439970

Grilo, C. M., White, M. A., Ivezaj, V., & Gueorguieva, R. (2020). Randomized controlled trial of behavioral weight loss and stepped care for binge-eating disorder: 12-month follow-up. *Obesity (Silver Spring, Md.), 28*(11), 2116–2124. https://doi.org/10.1002/oby.22957

Guarda, A. (2023). *What are eating disorders?* American Psychiatric Association. https://www.psychiatry.org/patients-families/eating-disorders/what-are-eating-disorders

Guarda, A. S., & Schreyer, C. C. (2010). Levels of care for eating disorders. In Herzog, D. B., Walsh, D. E., & Eddy, K. A. (Eds.), *Medical complications of eating disorders: A guide for professionals* (pp. 97–110). Massachusetts General Hospital and McGraw-Hill Medical.

Hagan, K. E., & Walsh, B. T. (2021). State of the art: The therapeutic approaches to bulimia nervosa. *Clinical Therapeutics, 43*(1), 40–49. DOI: 10.1016/j.clinthera.2020.10.012 PMID: 33358256

Hail, L., & Le Grange, D. (2018). Bulimia nervosa in adolescents: Prevalence and treatment challenges. *Adolescent Health, Medicine and Therapeutics, 9*, 11–16. DOI: 10.2147/AHMT.S135326 PMID: 29379324

Hamatani, S., Matsumoto, K., Ishibashi, T., Shibukawa, R., Honda, Y., Kosaka, H., Mizuno, Y., & Andersson, G. (2022). Development of a culturally adaptable internet-based cognitive behavioral therapy for Japanese women with bulimia nervosa. *Frontiers in Psychiatry, 13*(942936), 942936. Advance online publication. DOI: 10.3389/fpsyt.2022.942936 PMID: 36081468

Hartmann, A. S. (2015). Pica and rumination disorder. In *Encyclopedia of Feeding and Eating Disorders* (pp. 1–5). Springer., DOI: 10.1007/978-981-287-087-2_40-1

Haworth, J. J., Treadway, S., & Hobson, A. R. (2024). The prevalence of rumination syndrome and rumination disorder: A systematic review and meta-analysis. *Neurogastroenterology and Motility, 36*(7), e14793. DOI: 10.1111/nmo.14793 PMID: 38563201

Haynos, A. F., Watts, A. W., Loth, K. A., Pearson, C. M., & Neumark-Stzainer, D. (2016). Factors predicting an escalation of restrictive eating during adolescence. *The Journal of Adolescent Health, 59*(4), 391–396. DOI: 10.1016/j.jadohealth.2016.03.011 PMID: 27161416

Heafala, A., Ball, L., Rayner, J., & Mitchell, L. J. (2021). What role do dietitians have in providing nutrition care for eating disorder treatment? An integrative review. *Journal of Human Nutrition and Dietetics*, *34*(4), 724–735. DOI: 10.1111/jhn.12927 PMID: 34031923

Heo, Y.-A., & Duggan, S. T. (2017). Lisdexamfetamine: A review in binge eating disorder. *CNS Drugs*, *31*(11), 1015–1022. DOI: 10.1007/s40263-017-0477-1 PMID: 29134566

Hilbert, A., & van Dyck, Z. (2016). *Eating Disorders in Youth-Questionnaire. English version.* University of Leipzig: http://nbn-resolving.de/urn:nbn:de:bsz:15-qucosa-197246

Hilbert, A., Petroff, D., Herpertz, S., Pietrowsky, R., Tuschen-Caffier, B., Vocks, S., & Schmidt, R. (2019). Meta-analysis of the efficacy of psychological and medical treatments for binge-eating disorder. *Journal of Consulting and Clinical Psychology*, *87*(1), 91–105. DOI: 10.1037/ccp0000358 PMID: 30570304

Hilbert, A., Pike, K. M., Goldschmidt, A. B., Wilfley, D. E., Fairburn, C. G., Dohm, F. A., Walsh, T., & Striegel Weissman, R. (2014). Risk factors across the eating disorders. *Psychiatry Research*, *220*(1-2), 500–506. DOI: 10.1016/j.psychres.2014.05.054 PMID: 25103674

Hilbert, A., Zenger, M., Eichler, J., & Brähler, E. (2021). Psychometric evaluation of the Eating Disorders in Youth-Questionnaire when used in adults: Prevalence estimates for symptoms of avoidant/restrictive food intake disorder and population norms. *International Journal of Eating Disorders*, *54*(3), 399–408. DOI: 10.1002/eat.23424 PMID: 33283329

Izydorczyk, B., Sitnik-Warchulska, K., Lizińczyk, S., & Lipowska, M. (2020). Socio-cultural standards promoted by the mass media as predictors of restrictive and bulimic behavior. *Frontiers in Psychiatry*, *11*, 506. DOI: 10.3389/fpsyt.2020.00506 PMID: 32581880

Jakovina, T., Crnković Batista, M., Ražić Pavičić, A., Žurić Jakovina, I., & Begovac, I. (2018). Emotional dysregulation and attachment dimensions in female patients with bulimia nervosa. *Psychiatria Danubina*, *30*(1), 72–78. DOI: 10.24869/psyd.2018.72 PMID: 29546861

Jansen, P. W., de Barse, L. M., Jaddoe, V. W. V., Verhulst, F. C., Franco, O. H., & Tiemeier, H. (2017). Bi-directional associations between child fussy eating and parents' pressure to eat: Who influences whom? *Physiology & Behavior*, *176*, 101–106. DOI: 10.1016/j.physbeh.2017.02.015 PMID: 28215424

Jewell, T., Blessitt, E., Stewart, C., Simic, M., & Eisler, I. (2016). Family therapy for child and adolescent eating disorders: A critical review. *Family Process*, *55*(3), 577–594. DOI: 10.1111/famp.12242 PMID: 27543373

Kaplan, S. G., Arnold, E. M., Irby, M. B., Boles, K. A., & Skelton, J. A. (2014). Family systems theory and obesity treatment: Applications for clinicians. *Infant, Child & Adolescent Nutrition*, *6*(1), 24–29. DOI: 10.1177/1941406413516001 PMID: 24729831

Kaye, W. H., Fudge, J. L., & Paulus, M. (2009). New insights into symptoms and neurocircuit function of anorexia nervosa. *Nature Reviews. Neuroscience*, *10*(8), 573–584. DOI: 10.1038/nrn2682 PMID: 19603056

Kazdin, A. E., Fitzsimmons-Craft, E. E., & Wilfley, D. E. (2017). Addressing critical gaps in the treatment of eating disorders. *International Journal of Eating Disorders*, *50*(3), 170–189. DOI: 10.1002/eat.22670 PMID: 28102908

Keski-Rahkonen, A. (2021). Epidemiology of binge eating disorder: Prevalence, course, comorbidity, and risk factors. *Current Opinion in Psychiatry*, *34*(6), 525–531. DOI: 10.1097/YCO.0000000000000750 PMID: 34494972

Kozak, A., Czepczor-Bernat, K., Modrzejewska, J., Modrzejewska, A., Matusik, E., & Matusik, P. (2023). Avoidant/Restrictive Food Disorder (ARFID), food neophobia, other eating-related behaviours and feeding practices among children with autism spectrum disorder and in non-clinical sample: A preliminary study. *International Journal of Environmental Research and Public Health*, *20*(10), 5822. DOI: 10.3390/ijerph20105822 PMID: 37239549

Kurnik Mesarič, K., Damjanac, Ž., Debeljak, T., & Kodrič, J. (2024). Effectiveness of psychoeducation for children, adolescents and caregivers in the treatment of eating disorders: A systematic review. *European Eating Disorders Review*, *32*(1), 99–115. DOI: 10.1002/erv.3028 PMID: 37656835

Kutz, A. M., Marsh, A. G., Gunderson, C. G., Maguen, S., & Masheb, R. M. (2020). Eating disorder screening: A systematic review and meta-analysis of diagnostic test characteristics of the SCOFF. *Journal of General Internal Medicine*, *35*(3), 885–893. DOI: 10.1007/s11606-019-05478-6 PMID: 31705473

Lafrance Robinson, A., Dolhanty, J., & Greenberg, L. (2015). Emotion-focused family therapy for eating disorders in children and adolescents. *Clinical Psychology & Psychotherapy*, *22*(1), 75–82. DOI: 10.1002/cpp.1861 PMID: 23913713

Lakin, J., & Murphy, D. (2024). A pilot qualitative study of a person-centered approach to eating in women. *Person-Centered and Experiential Psychotherapies*, *23*(4), 512–530. https://doi.org/10.1080/14779757.2023.2273474

Landi, G., Simoni, E., Landi, I., Galeazzi, G. M., Moscara, M., Pighi, M., & Di Lorenzo, R. (2021). Therapeutic factors in a psychiatric group therapy: A preliminary validation of Therapeutic Factors Inventory-8, Italian version. *The Psychiatric Quarterly*, *92*(2), 523–536.

Latzer, Y., & Stein, D. (2019). Introduction: Novel perspectives on the psychology and psychotherapy of eating disorders. *Journal of Clinical Psychology*, *75*(8), 1369–1379. DOI: 10.1002/jclp.22786 PMID: 30995356

Lavender, K. R. (2020). Rebooting "failed" family-based treatment. *Frontiers in Psychiatry*, *11*(68), 68. Advance online publication. DOI: 10.3389/fpsyt.2020.00068 PMID: 32194444

Law, C., & Boisseau, C. L. (2019). Exposure and response prevention in the treatment of obsessive-compulsive disorder: Current perspectives. *Psychology Research and Behavior Management*, *12*, 1167–1174. DOI: 10.2147/PRBM.S211117

Linardon, J. (2018). Rates of abstinence following psychological or behavioral treatments for binge-eating disorder: Meta-analysis. *International Journal of Eating Disorders*, *51*(8), 785–797. DOI: 10.1002/eat.22897 PMID: 30058074

Linardon, J., Shatte, A., Messer, M., Firth, J., & Fuller-Tyszkiewicz, M. (2020). E-mental health interventions for the treatment and prevention of eating disorders: An updated systematic review and meta-analysis. *Journal of Consulting and Clinical Psychology*, *88*(11), 994–1007. DOI: 10.1037/ccp0000575 PMID: 32852971

Linehan, M. M., & Wilks, C. R. (2015). The course and evolution of dialectical behavior therapy. *American Journal of Psychotherapy*, *69*(2), 97–110. DOI: 10.1176/appi.psychotherapy.2015.69.2.97 PMID: 26160617

Liquori, S., Faidutti, G., Garzitto, M., Saetti, L., Bendotti, M., & Balestrieri, M. (2022). Efficacy of a group psychoeducation treatment in binge eating disorder: An open-label study. *Frontiers in Psychiatry*, *13*, 822282. Advance online publication. DOI: 10.3389/fpsyt.2022.822282 PMID: 35558418

Lloyd, S., Fleming, C., Schmidt, U., & Tchanturia, K. (2014). Targeting perfectionism in anorexia nervosa using a group-based cognitive behavioural approach: A pilot study. *European Eating Disorders Review*, *22*(5), 366–372. DOI: 10.1002/erv.2313 PMID: 25113819

Loeb, K. L., & Le Grange, D. (2009). Family-based treatment for adolescent eating disorders: Current status, new applications and future directions. *International Journal of Child and Adolescent Health*, *2*(2), 243–254. DOI: 10.1080/10640266.2010.509688 PMID: 20191109

Lucarelli, L., Sechi, C., Cimino, S., & Chatoor, I. (2018). Avoidant/Restrictive Food Intake Disorder: A longitudinal study of malnutrition and psychopathological risk factors from 2 to 11 years of age. *Frontiers in Psychology*, *9*, 1608. DOI: 10.3389/fpsyg.2018.01608 PMID: 30233458

MacCaughelty, C. R. (2023). Eating disorder mental health literacy: A national survey of clinical social workers in the United States. *Journal of Social Work : JSW*, *23*(2), 267–285. DOI: 10.1177/14680173221144217

Machado, B. C., Gonçalves, S. F., Martins, C., Hoek, H. W., & Machado, P. P. (2014). Risk factors and antecedent life events in the development of anorexia nervosa: A Portuguese case-control study. *European Eating Disorders Review*, *22*(4), 243–251. DOI: 10.1002/erv.2286 PMID: 24577737

Manlick, C. F., Cochran, S. V., & Koon, J. (2013). Acceptance and commitment therapy for eating disorders: Rationale and literature review. *Journal of Contemporary Psychotherapy*, *43*(2), 115–122. https://doi.org/10.1007/s10879-012-9223-7

Marcolini, F., Ravaglia, A., Tempia Valenta, S., Bosco, G., Marconi, G., De Ronchi, D., & Atti, A. R. (2024). Severe enduring anorexia nervosa (SE-AN) treatment options and their effectiveness: A review of literature. *Journal of Eating Disorders*, *12*(48), 48. Advance online publication. DOI: 10.1186/s40337-024-01006-y PMID: 38654374

Markowitz, J. C., & Weissman, M. M. (2004). Interpersonal psychotherapy: Principles and applications. *World Psychiatry; Official Journal of the World Psychiatric Association (WPA)*, *3*(3), 136–139. https://www.ncbi.nlm.nih.gov/pmc/articles/PMC1414693/ PMID: 16633477

Markowitz, J. C., & Weissman, M. M. (2012). Interpersonal psychotherapy: Past, present and future. *Clinical Psychology & Psychotherapy*, *19*(2), 99–105. DOI: 10.1002/cpp.1774 PMID: 22331561

Mateos-Agut, M., García-Alonso, I., De la Gándara-Martín, J. J., Vegas-Miguel, M. I., Sebastián-Vega, C., Sanz-Cid, B., Martínez-Villares, A., & Martín-Martínez, E. (2014). Family structure and eating behavior disorders. *Actas Españolas de Psiquiatría*, *42*(6), 267–280. https://actaspsiquiatria.es/index.php/actas/article/view/865 PMID: 25388769

Mercado, D., Robinson, L., Gordon, G., Werthmann, J., Campbell, I. C., & Schmidt, U. (2021). The outcomes of mindfulness-based interventions for obesity and binge eating disorder: A meta-analysis of randomised controlled trials. *Appetite*, *166*, 105464. DOI: 10.1016/j.appet.2021.105464

Merwin, R. M., Timko, C. A., Moskovich, A. A., Ingle, K. K., Bulik, C. M., & Zucker, N. L. (2011). Psychological inflexibility and symptom expression in anorexia nervosa. *Eating Disorders*, *19*(1), 62–82. https://doi.org/10.1080/10640266.2011.533606

Miao, D., Young, S. L., & Golden, C. D. (2015). A meta-analysis of pica and micronutrient status. *American Journal of Human Biology*, *27*(1), 84–93. DOI: 10.1002/ajhb.22598 PMID: 25156147

Micali, N., De Stavola, B., Ploubidis, G., Simonoff, E., Treasure, J., & Field, A. E. (2015). Adolescent eating disorder behaviours and cognitions: Gender-specific effects of child, maternal and family risk factors. *The British Journal of Psychiatry*, *207*(4), 320–327. DOI: 10.1192/bjp.bp.114.152371 PMID: 26206865

Miskovic-Wheatley, J., Bryant, E., Ong, S. H., Vatter, S., Le, A., Aouad, P., Barakat, S., Boakes, R., Brennan, L., Bryant, E., Byrne, S., Caldwell, B., Calvert, S., Carroll, B., Castle, D., Caterson, I., Chelius, B., Chiem, L., Clarke, S., & Maguire, S.National Eating Disorder Research Consortium. (2023). Eating disorder outcomes: Findings from a rapid review of over a decade of research. *Journal of Eating Disorders*, *11*(85), 85. Advance online publication. DOI: 10.1186/s40337-023-00801-3 PMID: 37254202

Moberg, L. T., Solvang, B., Sæle, R. G., & Myrvang, A. D. (2021). Effects of cognitive-behavioral and psychodynamic-interpersonal treatments for eating disorders: A meta-analytic inquiry into the role of patient characteristics and change in eating disorder-specific and general psychopathology in remission. *Journal of Eating Disorders*, *9*(74), 74. Advance online publication. DOI: 10.1186/s40337-021-00430-8 PMID: 34174942

Mohajer, R., Dick, S., Salinas, N. D., & Zolnikov, T. R. (2024). To eat, or not to eat? A psychoanalytic view on the food–parent. *British Journal of Psychotherapy*, *40*(4), 582–595. https://rave.ohiolink.edu/ejournals/article/4374142. DOI: 10.1111/bjp.12917

Moline, R., Hou, S., Chevrier, J., & Thomassin, K. (2021). A systematic review of the effectiveness of behavioural treatments for pica in youths. *Clinical Psychology & Psychotherapy*, *28*(1), 39–55. DOI: 10.1002/cpp.2491 PMID: 32628326

Monteleone, A. M., Fernandez-Aranda, F., & Voderholzer, U. (2019). Evidence and perspectives in eating disorders: A paradigm for a multidisciplinary approach. *World Psychiatry; Official Journal of the World Psychiatric Association (WPA)*, *18*(3), 369–370. DOI: 10.1002/wps.20687 PMID: 31496108

Monteleone, A., Pellegrino, F., Croatto, G., Carfagno, M., Hilbert, A., Treasure, J., Wade, T., Bulik, C. M., Zipfel, S., Hay, P., Schmidt, U., Castellini, G., Favaro, A., Fernandez-Aranda, F., Il Shin, J., Voderholzer, U., Ricca, V., Moretti, D., Busatta, D., & Solmi, M. (2022). Treatment of eating disorders: A systematic meta-review of meta- analyses and network meta-analyses. *Neuroscience and Biobehavioral Reviews*, *142*, 104857. DOI: 10.1016/j.neubiorev.2022.104857 PMID: 36084848

Monterubio, G. E., Fitzsimmons-Craft, E. E., & Wilfley, D. E. (2017). Interpersonal dysfunction as a risk factor for eating disorders. In Wade, T. (Ed.), *Encyclopedia of feeding and eating disorders* (pp. 1–4). Springer., DOI: 10.1007/978-981-287-104-6_29

Moreno, R., Buckelew, S. M., Accurso, E. C., & Raymond-Flesch, M. (2023). Disparities in access to eating disorders treatment for publicly-insured youth and youth of color: A retrospective cohort study. *Journal of Eating Disorders*, *11*(10), 10. Advance online publication. DOI: 10.1186/s40337-022-00730-7 PMID: 36694235

Morgan, J. F., Reid, F., & Lacey, J. H. (1999). The SCOFF questionnaire: Assessment of a new screening tool for eating disorders. *BMJ (Clinical Research Ed.)*, *319*(7223), 1467–1468. DOI: 10.1136/bmj.319.7223.1467 PMID: 10582927

Murphy, R., Straebler, S., Basden, S., Cooper, Z., & Fairburn, C. G. (2012). Interpersonal psychotherapy for eating disorders. *Clinical Psychology & Psychotherapy*, *19*(2), 150–158. DOI: 10.1002/cpp.1780 PMID: 22362599

Murphy, S., Russell, L., & Waller, G. (2005). Integrated psychodynamic therapy for bulimia nervosa and binge eating disorder: Theory, practice, and preliminary findings. *European Eating Disorders Review*, *13*(6), 383–391. DOI: 10.1002/erv.672

Nagata, J. M., Ganson, K. T., & Austin, S. B. (2020). Emerging trends in eating disorders among sexual and gender minorities. *Current Opinion in Psychiatry*, *33*(6), 562–567. DOI: 10.1097/YCO.0000000000000645 PMID: 32858597

National Association of Social Workers. (2021). *Code of ethics of the National Association of Social Workers.* https://www.socialworkers.org/About/Ethics/Code-of-Ethics/Code-of-Ethics-English/Social-Workers-Ethical-Responsibilities-to-Clients

National Association of Social Workers. (2025). *NASW standards for clinical social work in social work practice* (©2025). NASW Press. https://www.socialworkers.org/Practice/NASW-Practice-Standards-Guidelines/NASW-Standards-for-Clinical-Social-Work-in-Social-Work-Practice

National Association of Social Workers. (n.d.). *Evidence-based practice.* NASW. https://www.socialworkers.org/News/Research-Data/Social-Work-Policy-Research/Evidence-Based-Practice

National Eating Disorders Collaboration. (2022). *Eating disorders: A professional resource for general practitioners.* https://www.nedc.com.au/assets/NEDC-Resources/NEDC- Resource-GPs.pdf

Nicholls-Clow, R., Simmonds-Buckley, M., & Waller, G. (2024). Avoidant/restrictive food intake disorder: Systematic review and meta-analysis demonstrating the impact of study quality on prevalence rates. *Clinical Psychology Review*, *114*, 102502. DOI: 10.1016/j.cpr.2024.102502 PMID: 39298990

O'Connor, E., Garceau, C., Polhill, S., & Tasca, G. A. (2024). Evidence-based group therapy for eating disorders. *Group Dynamics*, *28*(3), 163–177. DOI: 10.1037/gdn0000221

Onnink, C. M., Konstantinidou, Y., Moskovich, A. A., Karekla, M. K., & Merwin, R. M. (2022). Acceptance and commitment therapy (ACT) for eating disorders: A systematic review of intervention studies and call to action. *Journal of Contextual Behavioral Science*, *26*, 11–28. https://doi.org/10.1016/j.jcbs.2022.08.005

Palavras, M. A., Hay, P., Mannan, H., da Luz, F. Q., Sainsbury, A., Touyz, S., & Claudino, A. M. (2021). Integrated weight loss and cognitive behavioural therapy (CBT) for the treatment of recurrent binge eating and high body mass index: A randomized controlled trial. *Eating and Weight Disorders*, *26*(1), 249–262.

Palombi, M. (2016). Separations: A personal account of Bowen Family Systems Theory. *Australian and New Zealand Journal of Family Therapy*, *37*(3), 327–339. DOI: 10.1002/anzf.1170

Pasquale, E. K., Boyar, A. M., & Boutelle, K. N. (2024). Reward and inhibitory control as mechanisms and treatment targets for binge eating disorder. *Current Psychiatry Reports*, *26*(9), 616–625. DOI: 10.1007/s11920-024-01534-z PMID: 39316228

Peckmezian, T., & Paxton, S. J. (2020). A systematic review of outcomes following residential treatment for eating disorders. *European Eating Disorders Review*, *28*(3), 246–259. DOI: 10.1002/erv.2733 PMID: 32196843

Penwell, T. E., Bedard, S. P., Eyre, R., & Levinson, C. A. (2024). Eating disorder treatment access in the United States: Perceived inequities among treatment seekers. *Psychiatric Services (Washington, D.C.)*, *75*(10), 944–952. Advance online publication. DOI: 10.1176/appi.ps.20230193 PMID: 38716514

Penwell, T. E., Smith, M., Ortiz, S. N., Brooks, G., & Thompson-Brenner, H. (2024). Traditional versus virtual partial hospital programme for eating disorders: Feasibility and preliminary comparison of effects. *European Eating Disorders Review*, *32*(2), 163–178. DOI: 10.1002/erv.3031 PMID: 37677002

Peterson, C. M., Kroon Van Diest, A. M., Mara, C. A., & Matthews, A. (2020). Dialectical behavioral therapy skills group as an adjunct to family-based therapy in adolescents with restrictive eating disorders. *Eating Disorders*, *28*(1), 67–79. DOI: 10.1080/10640266.2019.1568101 PMID: 30669955

Pietrabissa, G., Castelnuovo, G., Jackson, J. B., Rossi, A., Manzoni, G. M., & Gibson, P. (2019). Brief strategic therapy for bulimia nervosa and binge eating disorder: A clinical and research protocol. *Frontiers in Psychology*, *10*, 373. DOI: 10.3389/fpsyg.2019.00373 PMID: 30906269

Pike, K. M., So, M., Hilbert, A., Maekawa, H., Shimanouchi, T., Wilfley, D., Dohm, F., Fairburn, C. G., & Weissman, R. S. (2021). Risk factors for anorexia nervosa and bulimia nervosa in Japan and compared to a U.S. sample. *International Journal of Eating Disorders*, *54*(2), 155–167. DOI: 10.1002/eat.23442 PMID: 33355934

Pini, S., Abelli, M., Carpita, B., Dell'Osso, L., Castellini, G., Carmassi, C., & Ricca, V. (2016, July). Historical evolution of the concept of anorexia nervosa and relationships with orthorexia nervosa, autism, and obsessive–compulsive spectrum. *Neuropsychiatric Disease and Treatment*, *12*, 1651–1660. DOI: 10.2147/NDT.S108912 PMID: 27462158

Placek, C. D. (2017). Ethnomedical and sociocultural factors of pica substances in rural South India. *Ecology of Food and Nutrition*, *56*(3), 238–255. DOI: 10.1080/03670244.2017.1311255 PMID: 28418723

Qian, J., Wu, Y., Liu, F., Zhu, Y., Jin, H., Zhang, H., Wan, Y., Li, C., & Yu, D. (2022). An update on the prevalence of eating disorders in the general population: A systematic review and meta-analysis. *Eating and Weight Disorders*, *27*(2), 415–428. DOI: 10.1007/s40519-021-01162-z PMID: 33834377

Quiles Marcos, Y., Quiles Sebastián, M. J., Pamies Aubalat, L., Botella Ausina, J., & Treasure, J. (2013). Peer and family influence in eating disorders: A meta-analysis. *European Psychiatry : the Journal of the Association of European Psychiatrists*, *28*(4), 199–206. DOI: 10.1016/j.eurpsy.2012.03.005 PMID: 22944338

Rakhkovskaya, L. M., & Warren, C. S. (2014). Ethnic identity, thin-ideal internalization, and eating pathology in ethnically diverse college women. *Body Image*, *11*(4), 438–445. DOI: 10.1016/j.bodyim.2014.07.003 PMID: 25079012

Reyes-Rodriguez, M. L., Baucom, D. H., & Bulik, C. M. (2014). Culturally sensitive intervention for Latina women with eating disorders: A case study. *Revista Mexicana de Trastornos Alimentarios*, *5*(2), 136–146. DOI: 10.1016/S2007-1523(14)72009-9 PMID: 25598951

Ricca, V., Castellini, G., Mannucci, E., Lo Sauro, C., Ravaldi, C., Rotella, C. M., & Faravelli, C. (2010). Comparison of individual and group cognitive behavioral therapy for binge eating disorder: A randomized, three-year follow-up study. *Appetite*, *55*(3), 656–665. DOI: 10.1016/j.appet.2010.09.019 PMID: 20870000

Richards, J., Bang, N., Ratliff, E. L., Paszkowiak, M. A., Khorgami, Z., Khalsa, S. S., & Simmons, W. K. (2023). Successful treatment of binge eating disorder with the GLP-1 agonist semaglutide: A retrospective cohort study. *Obesity Pillars*, *7*, 100080. DOI: 10.1016/j.obpill.2023.100080 PMID: 37990682

Rizvi, S. L., Steffel, L. M., & Carson-Wong, A. (2013). An overview of dialectical behavior therapy for professional psychologists. *Professional Psychology, Research and Practice*, *44*(2), 73–80. DOI: 10.1037/a0029808

Rockwell, R. E., Boutelle, K., Trunko, M. E., Jacobs, M. J., & Kaye, W. H. (2011). An innovative short-term, intensive, family-based treatment for adolescent anorexia nervosa: Case series. *European Eating Disorders Review*, *19*(4), 362–367. DOI: 10.1002/erv.1094 PMID: 21308869

Rodgers, R. F., Berry, R., & Franko, D. L. (2018). Eating disorders in ethnic minorities: An update. *Current Psychiatry Reports*, *20*(10), 90. DOI: 10.1007/s11920-018-0938-3 PMID: 30155577

Roos, C. R., Sala, M., Kober, H., Vanzhula, I. A., & Levinson, C. A. (2021). Mindfulness-based interventions for eating disorders: The potential to mobilize multiple associative-learning change mechanisms. *International Journal of Eating Disorders*, *54*(9), 1601–1607. DOI: 10.1002/eat.23564

Ruchkin, V., Isaksson, J., Schwab-Stone, M., & Stickley, A. (2021). Prevalence and early risk factors for bulimia nervosa symptoms in inner-city youth: Gender and ethnicity perspectives. *Journal of Eating Disorders, 9*(1), 136. DOI: 10.1186/s40337-021-00479-5 PMID: 34674763

Russell, H., Aouad, P., Le, A., Marks, P., & Maloney, D.National Eating Disorder Research Consortium, Touyz, S., & Maguire, S. (2023). Psychotherapies for eating disorders: Findings from a rapid review. *Journal of Eating Disorders, 11*(1), 175. Advance online publication. DOI: 10.1186/s40337-023-00886-w

Sader, M., Weston, A., Buchan, K., Kerr-Gaffney, J., Gillespie-Smith, K., Sharpe, H., & Duffy, F. (2025). The co-occurrence of autism and avoidant/restrictive food intake disorder (ARFID): A prevalence-based meta-analysis. *International Journal of Eating Disorders, 58*(3), 473–488. Advance online publication. DOI: 10.1002/eat.24369 PMID: 39760303

Sasegbon, A., Hasan, S. S., Disney, B. R., & Vasant, D. H. (2022). Rumination syndrome: Pathophysiology, diagnosis and practical management. *Frontline Gastroenterology, 13*(5), 402–409. DOI: 10.1136/flgastro-2021-101856 PMID: 36046491

Schaefer, L. M., Burke, N. L., & Thompson, J. K. (2019). Thin-ideal internalization: How much is too much? *Eating and Weight Disorders, 24*(5), 933–937. DOI: 10.1007/s40519-018-0498-x PMID: 29549566

Shimshoni, Y., Silverman, W. K., & Lebowitz, E. R. (2020). SPACE-ARFID: A pilot trial of a novel parent-based treatment for avoidant/restrictive food intake disorder. *International Journal of Eating Disorders, 53*(10), 1623–1635. DOI: 10.1002/eat.23341 PMID: 33464594

Simpson, C. C., Towne, T. L., Karam, A. M., Donahue, J. M., Hadjeasgari, C. F., Rockwell, R., & Kaye, W. H. (2021). Predictors of stepping up to higher level of care among eating disorder patients in a partial hospitalization program. *Frontiers in Psychology, 12*, 667868. Advance online publication. DOI: 10.3389/fpsyg.2021.667868 PMID: 34366985

Slade, E., Keeney, E., Mavranezouli, I., Dias, S., Fou, L., Stockton, S., Saxon, L., Waller, G., Turner, H., Serpell, L., Fairburn, C. G., & Kendall, T. (2018). Treatments for bulimia nervosa: A network meta-analysis. *Psychological Medicine*, *48*(16), 2629–2636. DOI: 10.1017/S0033291718001071 PMID: 29729686

Smith, J. (2023). A call to shift theoretical orientation for eating disorder treatment in social work: Inside-out and outside-in. *Health & Social Work*, *48*(4), 281–284. DOI: 10.1093/hsw/hlad019 PMID: 37608569

Song, S., Stern, C. M., Deitsch, T., & Sala, M. (2023). Acculturation and eating disorders: A systematic review. *Eating and Weight Disorders*, *28*(39), 39. Advance online publication. DOI: 10.1007/s40519-023-01563-2 PMID: 37076614

Sonneville, K. R., & Lipson, S. K. (2018). Disparities in eating disorder diagnosis and treatment according to weight status, race/ethnicity, socioeconomic background, and sex among college students. *International Journal of Eating Disorders*, *51*(6), 518–526. DOI: 10.1002/eat.22846 PMID: 29500865

Sproch, L. E., & Anderson, K. P. (2019). Clinician-delivered teletherapy for eating disorders. *The Psychiatric Clinics of North America*, *42*(2), 243–252. DOI: 10.1016/j.psc.2019.01.008 PMID: 31046926

Steiger, H., & Booij, L. (2020). Eating disorders, heredity and environmental activation: Getting epigenetic concepts into practice. *Journal of Clinical Medicine*, *9*(5), 1332. DOI: 10.3390/jcm9051332 PMID: 32375223

Steinberg, D., Perry, T., Freestone, D., Bohon, C., Baker, J. H., & Parks, E. (2023). Effectiveness of delivering evidence-based eating disorder treatment via telemedicine for children, adolescents, and youth. *Eating Disorders*, *31*(1), 85–101. DOI: 10.1080/10640266.2022.2076334 PMID: 35695470

Steinhausen, H. C., Jakobsen, H., Helenius, D., Munk-Jørgensen, P., & Strober, M. (2015). A nation-wide study of the family aggregation and risk factors in anorexia nervosa over three generations. *International Journal of Eating Disorders*, *48*(1), 1–8. DOI: 10.1002/eat.22293 PMID: 24777686

Steward, T., Menchón, J. M., Jiménez-Murcia, S., Soriano-Mas, C., & Fernández-Aranda, F. (2017). Neural network alterations across eating disorders: A narrative review of fMRI studies. *Current Neuropharmacology, 15*(5), 1–13. DOI: 10.2174/1570159X15666171017111532 PMID: 29046154

Stice, E., Gau, J. M., Rohde, P., & Shaw, H. (2017). Risk factors that predict future onset of each *DSM–5* eating disorder: Predictive specificity in high-risk adolescent females. *Journal of Abnormal Psychology, 126*(1), 38–51. DOI: 10.1037/abn0000219 PMID: 27709979

Storch, E. A., & Guzick, A. G. (2025). *Childhood obsessive-compulsive and related disorders: Assessment and treatment*. Routledge.

Sue, D., Sue, D. W., Sue, D., & Sue, S. (2017). *Essentials of understanding abnormal behavior* (3rd ed.). Cengage.

Summers, F. (2024). *Object relations theories and psychopathology: A comprehensive text* (2nd ed.). Routledge.

Sysko, R., Glasofer, D. R., Hildebrandt, T., Klimek, P., Mitchell, J. E., Berg, K. C., Peterson, C. B., Wonderlich, S. A., & Walsh, B. T. (2015). The eating disorder assessment for DSM-5 (EDA-5): Development and validation of a structured interview for feeding and eating disorders. *International Journal of Eating Disorders, 48*(5), 452–463. DOI: 10.1002/eat.22388 PMID: 25639562

Telch, C. F., Agras, W. S., & Linehan, M. M. (2000). Group dialectical behavior therapy for binge-eating disorder: A preliminary, uncontrolled trial. *Behavior Therapy, 31*(3), 569–582. DOI: 10.1016/S0005-7894(00)80031-3

Thomas, B. R., Bowman, M. D., Sanchez, A., & Strohmeier, C. W. (2023). Parent treatment of complex pica in a teen with autism. *Behavioral Interventions, 38*(3), 611–624. DOI: 10.1002/bin.1956

Thomas, J. J., Becker, K. R., Breithaupt, L., Burton Murray, H., Jo, J. H., Kuhnle, M. C., Dreier, M. J., Harshman, S., Kahn, D. L., Hauser, K., Slattery, M., Misra, M., Lawson, E. A., & Eddy, K. T. (2021). Cognitive-behavioral therapy for adults with avoidant/restrictive food intake disorder. *Journal of Behavioral and Cognitive Therapy*, *31*(1), 47–55. DOI: 10.1016/j.jbct.2020.10.004 PMID: 34423319

Thomas, K., Dowd, C., & Broman-Fulks, J. J. (2017). Systematic desensitization. In Zeigler-Hill, V., & Shackelford, T. K. (Eds.), *Encyclopedia of personality and individual differences* (pp. 1–3). Springer., DOI: 10.1007/978-3-319-28099-8_952-1

Thomas, P. C., Curtis, K., Potts, H. W. W., Bark, P., Perowne, R., Rookes, T., & Rowe, S. (2024). Behavior change techniques within digital interventions for the treatment of eating disorders: Systematic review and meta-analysis. *JMIR Mental Health*, *11*, e57577. DOI: 10.2196/57577 PMID: 39088817

Tian, Z. (2023). Understanding and treating eating disorders in a psychoanalytic approach. *Proceedings of the 4th International Conference on Educational Innovation and Philosophical Inquiries*. https://doi.org/ DOI: 10.54254/2753-7048/18/20231276

Tournayre, L., Balbinotti, M. A. A., & Monthuy-Blanc, J. (2024). Some hope for a dimensional assessment? A critical review of psychometric validated (semi-)structured interview to assess eating disorders. *European Eating Disorders Review*, *32*(6), 1138–1156. DOI: 10.1002/erv.3115 PMID: 38873932

Trombetta, T., Bottaro, D., Paradiso, M. N., Rocchi, M. B. L., Polselli, G. M., & Biondi, M. (2024). Psychodynamic group therapy for eating disorders: A narrative review. *Journal of Contemporary Psychotherapy*, *54*(3), 253–264. DOI: 10.1007/s10879-023-09614-6

Ulfvebrand, S., Birgegård, A., Norring, C., Högdahl, L., & von Hausswolff-Juhlin, Y. (2015). Psychiatric comorbidity in women and men with eating disorders: Results from a large clinical database. *Psychiatry Research*, *230*(2), 294–299. DOI: 10.1016/j.psychres.2015.09.008 PMID: 26416590

Van Dyne, A., Washington, N., Villodas, M., & Cronan, T. (2023). Racial/ethnic differences in anorexia and bulimia diagnoses among U.S. college students. *Eating Behaviors*, *50*, 101779. DOI: 10.1016/j.eatbeh.2023.101779 PMID: 37418803

Wetchler, J. L., & Hecker, L. L. (2015). *An introduction to marriage and family therapy* (2nd ed.). Routledge.

Wetzler, S., Hackmann, C., Peryer, G., Clayman, K., Friedman, D., Saffran, K., Silver, J., Swarbrick, M., Magill, E., & Magill, E. (2020). A framework to conceptualize personal recovery from eating disorders: A systematic review and qualitative meta-synthesis of perspectives from individuals with lived experience. *International Journal of Eating Disorders*, *53*(8), 1188–1203. https://doi.org/10.1002/eat.23260

White, M., Thomas, A., Aston, M., & Joy, P. (2024). "It's beautiful and it's messy and it's tragic": Exploring the role of compassion in the eating disorder recovery processes of 2S/LGBTQ+ Canadians. *Journal of Eating Disorders*, *12*(23), 23. Advance online publication. DOI: 10.1186/s40337-024-00981-6 PMID: 38326869

Williams, F., Gibbs, S., & Addo, A. S. (2022). The assessment and management of pica in people with intellectual disability. *BJPsych Advances*, *28*(6), 391–400. DOI: 10.1192/bja.2022.24

Willmott, E., Dickinson, R., Hall, C., Sadikovic, K., Wadhera, E., Micali, N., Trompeter, N., & Jewell, T. (2024). A scoping review of psychological interventions and outcomes for avoidant and restrictive food intake disorder (ARFID). *International Journal of Eating Disorders*, *57*(1), 27–61. DOI: 10.1002/eat.24073 PMID: 37876356

Wonderlich, S. A., Bulik, C. M., Schmidt, U., Steiger, H., & Hoek, H. W. (2020). Achieving global impact: Increasing access to care and reducing the burden of eating disorders. *International Journal of Eating Disorders*, *53*(8), 1303–1312. DOI: 10.1002/eat.23283 PMID: 32359125

Yamamiya, Y., & Stice, E. (2024). Risk factors that predict future onset of anorexia nervosa, bulimia nervosa, binge eating disorder, and purging disorder in adolescent girls. *Behavior Therapy*, *55*(4), 712–723. DOI: 10.1016/j.beth.2023.10.002 PMID: 38937045

Zanella, E., & Lee, E. (2022). Integrative review on psychological and social risk and prevention factors of eating disorders including anorexia nervosa and bulimia nervosa: Seven major theories. *Heliyon*, *8*(11), e11422. DOI: 10.1016/j.heliyon.2022.e11422 PMID: 36406673

Zerbe, K. (2015). Psychodynamic theory of eating disorders. In Smolak, L., & Levine, M. P. (Eds.), *The Wiley handbook of eating disorders*. Wiley-Blackwell., DOI: 10.1002/9781118574089.ch20

Zhang, K., Xie, Q., Fan, C., Hu, X., Lei, J., Kong, J., Liang, M., Luo, J., & Li, X. (2024). The effectiveness of interpersonal psychotherapy versus cognitive behavioural therapy for eating disorders: A systematic review and meta-analysis. *Clinical Psychology & Psychotherapy*, *31*(1), e2953. DOI: 10.1002/cpp.2953

Zhang, Z. J., Lo, H. H. M., Ng, S. M., Mak, W. W. S., Wong, S. Y. S., Hung, K. S. Y., Lo, C. S. L., Wong, J. O. Y., Lui, S. S. Y., Lin, E., Siu, C. M. W., Yan, E. W. C., Chan, S. H. W., Yip, A., Poon, M. F., Wong, G. O. C., Mak, J. W. H., Tam, H. S. W., Tse, I. H. H., & Leung, B. F. H. (2023). The effects of a mindfulness-based family psychoeducation intervention for the caregivers of young adults with first-episode psychosis: A randomized controlled trial. *International Journal of Environmental Research and Public Health*, *20*(2), 1018. https://doi.org/10.3390/ijerph20021018

Zimmerman, J., & Fisher, M. (2017). Avoidant/restrictive food intake disorder (ARFID). *Current Problems in Pediatric and Adolescent Health Care*, *47*(4), 95–103. DOI: 10.1016/j.cppeds.2017.02.005 PMID: 28532967

Zipfel, S., Giel, K. E., Bulik, C. M., Hay, P., & Schmidt, U. (2015). Anorexia nervosa: Aetiology, assessment, and treatment. *The Lancet. Psychiatry*, *2*(12), 1099–1111. https://www.thelancet.com/journals/lanpsy/article/PIIS2215-0366(15)00356-9/fulltext. DOI: 10.1016/S2215-0366(15)00356-9 PMID: 26514083

About the Author

Jennifer Schulz (previously Jacobsen) is a professor in the Psychology, Social Work, Criminal Justice, and Sociology Department at Ashland University in North Central Ohio. She teaches courses on human rights, social welfare, human behavior, abnormal psychology, research methods, and social policy. She maintains an active clinical license and performs contract work as a crisis therapist, in addition to providing writing and consultation services related to evidence-based practices in social work and psychology. Her research interests focus on eating disorders and other mental health topics. Dr. Schulz taught for five years at Mount Vernon Nazarene University before accepting her current position at Ashland University. She holds a Doctor of Philosophy in Psychology from National University and a Master of Social with with an emphasis on mental health and substance abuse counseling from The Ohio State University.

Index

A

B

C

U

W

www.ingramcontent.com/pod-product-compliance
Lightning Source LLC
LaVergne TN
LVHW080859300926
849162LV00003B/479